Oliver Sacks was born in London in 1933 and trained at the
Middlesex Hospital. Following a period of research in
neurochemistry and neurophysiology, he returned to clinical work,
interesting himself particularly in migraine, mental illness,
behavioural development and the care of post-encephalitic patients
described in his book *Awakenings*. He is Professor of Clinical
Neurology at the Albert Einstein College of Medicine, New
York, and consultant neurologist to a number of New York
Hospitals. Dr Sacks's other books *Awakenings*, *A Leg to Stand on*,
and *The Man Who Mistook His Wife for a Hat* are published by
Picador.

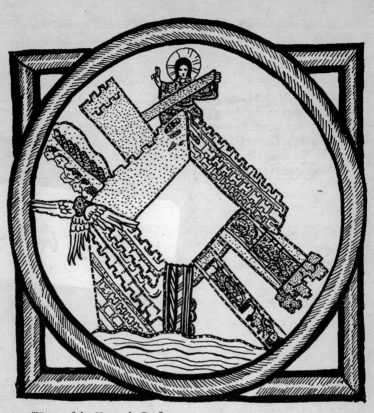

"Vision of the Heavenly City"
From a MS of Hildegard's *Scivias*, written at Bingen about 1180.
This figure is a reconstruction from several versions of migrainous origin
(see chapter 3, and *figure 6*).

Migraine
Understanding a
Common Disorder expanded and updated

Oliver Sacks

Pan Books

To my parents

Publisher's Note
Recent published articles referred to on pages
88, 90 and 92 are now available in
The Man Who Mistook His Wife for a Hat
(Picador, 1986)

First published in the USA by
University of California Press
This Edition published in Great Britain by
Pan Books Ltd, Cavaye Place, London SW10 9PG

9 8 7 6 5 4 3 2 1

© Oliver Sacks, 1985
ISBN 0 330 30015 6

Printed and bound in Great Britain by
Cox & Wyman Ltd, Reading

Contents

Socrates, in Plato, would prescribe no Physick for Charmides' headache till first he had eased his troublesome mind; body and soul must be cured together, as head and eyes . . .

—Robert Burton, *The Anatomy of Melancholy*

Foreword

The affliction of migraine has been described for at least the past 2,000 years; and no doubt every generation of modern man, with his history of perhaps 250,000 years, has its experience of this constellation of disorders. Yet it is a very common opinion of the public and the medical profession that little is known about migraine and even less to be done about it. Only in 1970 have arrangements been made for a clinic to deal with migraine to be set up in the City of London.

It is true that migraine is listed in textbooks of medicine and especially of neurology, but usually rather briefly among other intermittent disorders such as epilepsy and neuralgia. The common attitude is that migraine is merely a form of mainly nondisabling headache which occupies far more of a busy doctor's time than its importance warrants. Some of the accompaniments, such as vomiting and visual disturbances, are well recognized; sometimes to the extent that a diagnosis of migraine will be made only when a set pattern of visual upset, headache, and vomiting occurs in regular order. Some tablets and the current inelegant cliché of "learning to live with it" are advised by the physician, who hopes that he will not be on duty the next time the patient comes for advice. Because of the lack of full comprehension of the complexities and variabilities of a condition which is in every way fascinating in its phenomenology, many doctors are only too pleased when a patient, in desperation, takes himself off to the practitioners of "fringe medicine," almost hoping that the results will be both disastrous and very costly.

Is the medical profession entirely at fault? Does the name of an authoritative or "definitive" textbook spring to mind? Are there numerous well-equipped and properly organized centers where the condition may be studied? Are there extensive statistics about the whole problem, such as there are for, say, industrial accidents, bronchial carcinoma, or measles? Did we have as students a single lecture on migraine, and did anyone tell us that migraine is not just a tiresome form of occasional headache which someone else rather boringly suffers from? Almost certainly not; and the awareness that migraine is an expression of the genetics, personality, and way of life of an individual is only very recently being proclaimed.

Another remarkably neglected aspect of the migrainous process is the disorder of physiology which it expresses. In no other condition may we find the complete physiological experiment in a human being which the migrainous attack provides. We see, we may feel ourselves, the gradual disintegration of function of the normal person, exactly as we do in a case of stroke or of brain tumor; but without the disaster of the permanent disability. Within a few minutes or an hour or so the attack is past; the symptoms and signs, which may include those of dysphasia and hemiplegia, double vision, vertigo, vomiting, bowel disturbance, water balance changes, personality disorders, have vanished. However, few studies have been carried out under these circumstances; and research, such as it is, is more likely to have been carried out on more or less anesthetized animals, who probably do not have migraine as we know of it.

To redress this imbalance of interest, experience, physiological knowledge and therapeutic enterprise, we need a synoptic work which sets out for us all the whole scope of the migrainous spacetime continuum, the lifelong pattern of ever-changing features and factors which the patient with migraine both suffers and creates. His social circle, his work associates, and especially his physicians are inseparable elements in this continuum.

Dr. Oliver Sacks has undertaken the task of providing the general view which has for so long been lacking. In an immensely energetic act of clinical scholarship, he has brought together virtually all the features of modern knowledge on the subject of migraine. It is an interesting academic exercise for the neurologist to try and detect the omission of some minor point which he believes that he, almost alone, may have noted. It is extremely hard to find any such omission.

Let us hope that this work will achieve full success from its determination to illumine the grand scheme of migraine. Any such success must have immense benefits to individual patients, and also to both medical practitioners and society in general.

William Gooddy

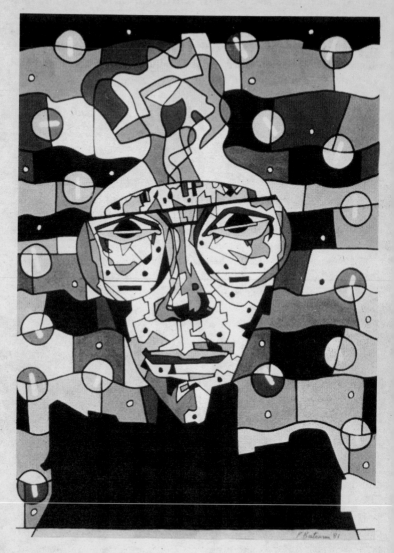

Many perceptual alterations may occur in migraine. The strangest
and profoundest is *mosaic vision* (pp. 85-87), here shown
in a painting done by a migraine sufferer asked to paint what he
experienced during his attacks. (Courtesy British Migraine
Association and Boehringer Ingelheim Limited.)

Preface to New Edition

Fifteen years have passed since *Migraine* was first published. In this new edition I have made certain additions and changes. I have added a number of new observations and reflections, in the text or as addenda and footnotes; and, at the end, a Glossary of some of the technical terms occasionally used.

I have revised Part 3, The Basis of Migraine, avoiding the lengthy academic discussion to be found in the original edition. What remains is, I think, clearer, and more directly related to the experience and needs of ordinary patients.

I have rather radically altered the perspective and tone of Part 4, which deals with the treatment of migraine, so that it is more directly addressed to the patient himself. At the time of writing the original edition, my experience was especially with "intractable" migraine, those (rather rare) patients who are unresponsive to straightforward simple measures, and so require intensive and special medical care. Since 1970, I have seen numbers of patients with more 'ordinary' migraine, and have become much more optimistic about the effectiveness of self-help and self-care. For this reason, I have somewhat expanded the *Conclusions*, making them broader and deeper, and more personal, and added at the end an Epilogue, "The Long Road."

The last fifteen years have seen advances in our knowledge of the causes of migraine, and of medications and other measures that promise more relief: these find their place, now, in this edition for the eighties.

1985   *O. W. S.*

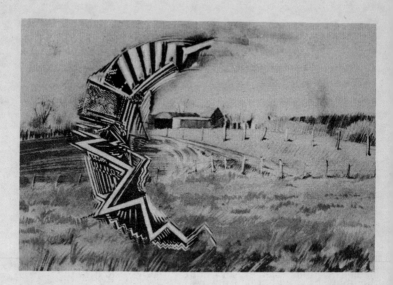

The most common visual alteration is a *scintillating scotoma* (Chapter 3), painted here by another migraine sufferer. (Courtesy British Migraine Association and Boehringer Ingelheim Limited.)

Preface to Original Edition

When I saw my first migraine patient, I thought of migraine as a peculiar type of headache, no more and no less. As I saw more patients, it became apparent to me that headache was never the sole feature of a migraine, and, later still, that it was not even a necessary feature of all migraines. I was moved, therefore, to inquire further into a subject which appeared to retreat before me, growing more complex, less capable of circumscription, and less intelligible, the more I learned of it. I delved into the literature of the subject, submerged, and then reemerged, more knowledgeable in some ways but more confused in others. I returned to my patients whom I found more instructive than any book. And after I had seen a thousand migraine patients, I saw that the subject made *sense*.

I was at first disconcerted, but later delighted, at the complexity of the histories I received. Here was something which could pass, in a few minutes, from the subtlest disorders of perception, speech, emotion and thought, to every conceivable vegetative symptom. Every patient with classical migraine opened out, as it were, into an entire encyclopedia of neurology.

I was recalled from my neurological preoccupation by the suffering of my patients and their appeals for help. Some patients I could help with drugs, and some with the magic of attention and interest. The most severely afflicted patients defeated my therapeutic endeavors until I started to inquire minutely and persistently into their emotional lives. It now became apparent to me that many migraine attacks were drenched in emotional significance, and could not be usefully considered, let alone treated, unless their emotional antecedents and effects were exposed in detail.

I thus found it necessary to employ a sort of continuous double-vision, simultaneously envisaging migraine as a *structure* whose forms were implicit in the repertoire of the nervous system, and as a *strategy* which might be employed to any emotional, or indeed biological, end.

I have endeavored, in the composition of this book, to keep these two perspectives constantly in view, portraying migraines as both physical and symbolic events. Part 1 is devoted to describing the forms of migraine attacks as experienced by the patient and observed by the physician. Part 2 is concerned with the many circumstances—physical, physiological, and psychological—which may provoke isolated or repeated migraine attacks. Part 3 considers the physiological mechanisms of the migraine attack, and discusses the biological and psychological roles which migraines, and certain allied disorders, may fill. Part 4 is concerned with the therapeutic approach to migraine, and forms both a corollary and a supplement to the preceding portions of the book.

I have used simple language wherever possible, and technical language wherever necessary. Although the first two parts of this work are primarily descriptive, in contrast to the third part which is explanatory and speculative, I have at all times moved freely, perhaps too freely, between the statement of facts and the questioning of their meaning. If the frame of reference is steadily broadened, its expansion is demanded by the many, various, and sometimes very strange facts we are forced to consider.

I entertain the hope that three groups of readers may find something of interest in this book. First, sufferers from migraine, and their physicians, who seek an intelligible account of what migraine is, and how to treat it. Secondly, students and investigators of migraine, who may be assured of finding a detailed, if somewhat discursive, reference book on the subject. Lastly, general readers of a speculative turn of mind (not necessarily medical men!), who are invited to see in migraine something that has countless familiar analogies in human and animal functioning, a model that illuminates the entire range of psychophysiological reactions, by reminding us, again and again, of the absolute continuity of mind and body.

1970   *O. W. S.*

Acknowledgments

My first debt is to my many and long-suffering migraine patients, to whom I owe the possibility of this book. They have provided me with the clinical reality from which all observations were derived, and against which every idea has had to be tested. In a very real sense, therefore, this is *their* book.

I owe to many close (and frequently migrainous) friends a variety of ideas and criticisms offered during the course of vigorous discussions on and around the subject of migraine. A special joy, since publication of the original edition, has been correspondence with Dr. Walter Alvarez, Dr. J. C. Steele, Professor G. W. Bruyn and many other colleagues eminent for their contributions to our understanding of migraine. My brother, Mr. Michael Sacks, has greatly assisted me in the preparation of a bibliography, a glossary, and other necessities; my parents and other relatives (also migrainous, for the most part) have reacted candidly and constructively when compelled to listen to each chapter as it was written.

I am grateful to Constable and Company for permission to reproduce five diagrams from C. Singer's *From Magic to Science* (frontispiece and *figure six*); and to the American Medical Association for permission to reproduce two diagrams from an article by K. Lashley published in the *Archives for Neurology and Psychiatry* of 1941. These, and other diagrams from original sources, have been redrawn and somewhat modified.

I am particularly indebted to Dr. William Gooddy, who was kind enough to read the original version of my manuscript, to encourage the hope of its publication, and to suggest many valuable additions and emendations. Since receiving his friendly advice on the original work, I have, after a famous precedent, suppressed a third, added a third, and altered a third.

I must acknowledge the continued encouragement and expert assistance of my editor, Miss Jean Cunningham, the skill of Mrs. Audrey Besterman, who drew or redrew the many figures in this volume, and the great courtesy with which Messrs. Faber and Faber treated me throughout. Finally, I must acknowledge my gratitude to the University of California Press for all their encouragement and help in bringing out this enlarged, new edition of *Migraine*.

Historical Introduction

Migraine affects a substantial minority of the population, occurs in all civilizations, and has been recognized since the dawn of recorded history. If it was a scourge, or an encouragement, to Caesar, Paul, Kant, and Freud, it is also a daily fact of life to anonymous millions who suffer in secrecy and silence. Its forms and symptoms, as Burton remarked of melancholy, are "irregular, obscure, various, so infinite, Proteus himself is not so diverse." Its nature and causes puzzled Hippocrates, and have been the subject of argument for two thousand years.

The major clinical characteristics of migraine—its periodicity, its relation to character and circumstance, its physical and emotional symptoms—had all been clearly recognized by the second century of our era. Thus Aretaeus describes it, under the name of Heterocrania:

And in certain cases the whole head is pained, and the pain is sometimes on the right, and sometimes on the left side, or the forehead, or the fontanelle; and such attacks shift their place during the same day. . . . This is called Heterocrania, an illness by no means mild. . . . It occasions unseemly and dreadful symptoms . . . nausea; vomiting of bilious matters; collapse of the patient . . . there is much torpor, heaviness of the head, anxiety; and life becomes a burden. For they flee the light; the darkness soothes their disease; nor can they bear readily to look upon or hear anything pleasant. . . . The patients are weary of life and wish to die.

While his contemporary Pelops described and named the sensory symptoms which might precede an epilepsy (the aura), Aretaeus

1

observed the analogous symptoms which inaugurated certain migraines:

. . . flashes of purple or black colors before the sight, or all mixed together, so as to exhibit the appearance of a rainbow expanded in the heavens.

Fourteen hundred years elapsed between the observations of Aretaeus and the treatises of Alexander Trallianus. Throughout this period repeated observations confirmed and elaborated the terse description of Aretaeus, while reiterating, unquestioned, the theories of antiquity concerning its nature. The terms *heterocrania, holocrania,* and *hemicrania* struggled with one another for many centuries; hemicrania ousted its rivals, and has finally evolved, through an immense number of transliterations, to the migraine or megrim we speak of today.* The terms *sick-headache, bilious-headache (cephalgia biliosa),* and *blind-headache* have been in popular use for many centuries.

Two categories of theory have dominated medical thinking on the nature of migraine since the time of Hippocrates; both were still a matter of serious dispute at the end of the eighteenth century, and both, variously transformed, command wide popular assent today. It is, therefore, no work of supererogation, but one of the greatest relevance to trace the evolution of these two classical theories. We will speak of the humoral theory and the sympathetic theory.

An excess of yellow or black bile, it was supposed, could occasion not only a liverish feeling, a black humor, or a jaundiced view of life, but the bilious vomiting and gastric upset of a sick-headache.**

---

*The *Oxford English Dictionary* provides an exhaustive list of these transliterations and their usages. A mere fraction of these may be cited: Mygrane, Megryne, Migrane, Mygrame, Migrym, Myegrym, Midgrame, Midgramme, Mygrim, Magryme, Maigram, Meigryme, Megrym, Megrome, Meagrim . . . The first use of any of these terms in English was apparently in the fourteenth century: "the mygrame and other euyll passyons of the head." The French term *Migraine* was in use a century earlier.

**A variant of the humoral theory attributed migraines to the spleen and splenetic humors. Pope (himself an inveterate migraineur) has preserved this concept in his description of the Cave of Spleen in *The Rape of the Lock:*

> Where screen'd in shades from day's detested glare,
> Spleen sighs for ever on her pensive bed,
> Pain at her side, and *megrim* at her head.

The essence of this theory, and of the form of treatment which it implies, is precisely expressed by Alexander Trallianus:

If therefore headache frequently arises on account of a superfluity of bilious humor, the cure of it must be affected by means of remedies which purge and draw away the bilious humor.

Purging and drawing away the bilious humor—in this lies the historical justification of innumerable derivative theories and treatments, many of them practiced at the present day. The stomach and bowel may become laden with bilious humors: hence the immemorial use of emetics, laxatives, cathartics, purgatives, and the like. Fatty foods draw bilious humors to the stomach, therefore the diet of the migraineur must be sparse and ascetic. Thus, the puritanical Fothergill, a lifelong sufferer from migraine, considered the following especially dangerous:

Melted butter, fat meats, spices, meat pies, hot buttered toast, and malt liquors when strong and hoppy.

Similarly, it has always been considered, and is still so held, that constipation (i.e., retention of bilious humors in the bowel) may provoke or prelude an attack of migraine. Similarly, bilious humors might be reduced at their source (a variety of liver pills is still recommended for migraine), or diminished if their concentration in the blood became too high (blood-letting was particularly recommended in the sixteenth and seventeenth centuries as a cure for migraine). It is not, perhaps, unduly farfetched to regard current chemical theories of the origin of migraine as intellectual descendants of the ancient humoral doctrines.

Contemporary in origin with the humoral theories, and evolving concurrently with them, have been a variety of "sympathetic" theories. These hold that migraine has a peripheral origin in one or more of the viscera (the stomach, the bowel, the uterus, etc.), from which it is propagated about the body by a special form of internal, visceral communication; this occult form of communication, hidden from and below the transactions of consciousness, was termed *sympathy* by the Greeks, and *consensus* by the Romans, and was conceived to be of particular importance in connecting the head and the viscera (mirum inter caput et viscera commercium).

The classical notions of sympathy were revived and given a more exact form by Thomas Willis. Willis had come to reject the Hippocratic notions of hysteria as arising from the physical trajectory of the womb about the body, and instead came to visualize the uterus as *radiating* the phenomenon of hysteria through an infinitude of minute pathways about the body. He extended this concept to the transmission of a migraine throughout the body and of many other paroxysmal disorders.

Willis set out, three centuries ago, to review the entire domain of nervous disorders (*De Anima Brutorum*), and in the course of this work included a section ("De Cephalalgia") which must be considered as the first modern treatise on migraine, and the first decisive advance since the time of Aretaeus. He organized a vast mass of medieval observations and speculations on the subjects of migraine, epilepsy, and other paroxysmal reactions, and added to these clinical observations which were extraordinary in their accuracy and sobriety. Consulted on one occasion by a lady with a headache, he has passed down to us the following incomparable description of migraine:

Some years since I was sent for to visit a most noble Lady, for above twenty years sick with almost a continual Headach, at first intermitting . . . she was extremely punished with this Disease. Growing well of a Feavour before she was twelve years old, she became obnoxious to pains in the Head, which were wont to arise, sometimes of their own accord, and more often upon very light occasion. This sickness being limited to no one place of the Head, troubled her sometimes on one side, sometimes on the other, and often thorow the whole compass of the Head. During the fit (which rarely ended under a day and a night's space, and often held for two, three, or four days) she was impatient of light, speaking, noise, or of any motion, sitting upright in her Bed, the Chamber made dark, she would talk to nobody, nor take any sleep, or sustenance. At length about the declination of the fit, she was wont to lye down with a heavy and disturbed sleep, from which awakening she found herself better. . . . Formerly, the fits came not but occasionally, and seldom under twenty days of a month, but afterwards they came more often; and lately she was seldom free.

Willis, discussing this case, shows himself fully aware of the many predisposing, exciting and accessory causes of such attacks: "An evil or weak constitution of the parts . . . sometimes innate and hereditary . . . an irritation in some distant member or viscera . . . changes of season, atmospheric states, the great aspects of the sun and moon, violent passions, and errors in diet." He was well aware, also, that migraine, though frequently intolerable, is benign:

But although this Distemper most greviously afflicting this noble Lady, above twenty years . . . having pitched its tents near the confines of the Brain, had so long besieged its regal tower, yet it had not taken it; for the sick Lady, being free from a Vertigo, swimming in the Head, Convulsive Distempers, and any Soporiferous symptoms, found the chief faculties of her soul sound enough.

The other classical concept revived by Willis was that of *idiopathy*, a tendency to periodic and sudden explosions in the nervous system. Thus the migrainous nervous system, or the epileptic nervous system, could be detonated at any time, by a variety of influences—physical or emotional—and the remotest effects of the explosion were conveyed throughout the body by sympathy, by presumed sympathetic nerves whose existence Willis himself could only infer.

Sympathetic theories were particularly favored and elaborated in the eighteenth century. Tissot, observing that stomach disorders might precede and apparently inaugurate a migraine headache, and that vomiting could rapidly bring the entire attack to a close, suggests:

It is then most probable that a focus of irritation is formed little by little in the stomach, and that when it has reached a certain point, the irritation is sufficient to give rise to acute pains in all the ramifications of the supraorbital nerve. . . .

Contemporary with Tissot, and also lending the weight of his authority to such sympathetic theories, was Robert Whytt; observing "the vomiting that generally accompanies inflammation of the womb; the nausea, the disordered appetite, that follows conception . . . the headache, the heat and pains in the back, the intestinal colic suffered when the time of the menstrual flow approaches," Whytt pictures the human body (in Foucault's eloquent paraphrase) as riddled, from one extremity to another, by obscure but strangely direct paths of sympathy: paths which could transmit the phenomena of a migraine, or a hysteria, from their visceral origins.

It is important to note that the finest clinical observers of the eighteenth century—Tissot (who wrote voluminously on migraine, and whose 1790 treatise was the true successor of Willis' "De Cephalalgia"), Whytt, Cheyne, Cullen, Sydenham, and others— made no arbitrary distinctions between physical and emotional symptoms: all had to be considered together, as integral parts of "nervous disorders." Thus Robert Whytt brings together, as intimate and interrelated symptoms

an extraordinary sensation of cold and heat, of pains in several parts of the body; syncopes and vaporous convulsions; catalepsy and tetanus; gas in the stomach and intestines . . . vomiting of black matter; a sudden and abundant flow of clear pale urine . . . palpitations of the heart; variations in the pulse; *periodic headaches;* vertigo and nervous spells . . . depression, despair . . . madness, nightmares or incubi.

This central belief, this concept of the inseparable unity of body and mind, was fractured at the start of the nineteenth century. The "nervous disorders" of Willis and Whytt were rigidly divided into "organic" versus "functional," and as rigidly partitioned between neurologists and mental pathologists; Liveing and Jackson, it is true, did portray migraine as an indivisible psychophysiological entity without internal divisions, but their views were exceptional and against the bias of their century.

Superb descriptions of migraine appeared in great numbers with the opening of the nineteenth century, almost all of which had a vividness which seems to have vanished from the medical literature. Looking back on the riches of this older literature, one is tempted to imagine that every physician of note either had migraine or made it his business to describe the phenomenon: included in this galaxy of names are those of Heberden and Wollaston, in the first decade of the century, Abercrombie, Piorry and Parry in its second and third decades, Romberg, Symonds, Hall, and Möllendorf around the middle of the century; brilliant descriptions were also provided by a number of non-medical men, among whom the astronomers Herschel and the Airies (father and son) were preeminent.

Almost all of these descriptions, however, dwelt on the *physical* aspects of migraine attacks, while neglecting their emotional components, antecedents, and uses. The theories of the nineteenth century, likewise, lacked the generality of the earlier doctrines, and were usually concerned with very specific mechanical etiologies of one type or another. Vascular theories were very popular, whether these envisaged general plethora, cerebral congestion, or specific dilatations and constrictions of the cranial vessels. Local factors were given great weight: swelling of the pituitary gland, inflammation in the eyes, and so forth. Hereditary "taint" and masturbation were also inculpated toward the middle of the century (they had also been summoned to explain epilepsy and insanity), and in such theories—as in later theories of autointoxication, infective foci, etc.—an anachronistic quality is apparent, for the mode of action was ostensibly physical, but covertly and implicitly moral.

Homage must be singled out for the remarkable Victorian masterpiece, Edward Liveing's treatise *On Megrim, Sick-Headache and Some Allied Disorders*, which was composed between 1863 and 1865, but only published in 1873. Bringing to his subject the acumen and learning of a Gowers, and the imaginative depth and range of a Hughlings Jackson, Liveing encompassed and ordered the entire range of migrainous experience, and its place amid an immense surrounding field of "allied and metamorphic disorders." As Hughlings Jackson utilized the phenomena of epilepsy to visualize the evolution and dissolution of hierarchically organized functions in the nervous system, so Liveing performed a comparable task using the data of migraine. Historical depth and generality of approach must be the justifications of any medical essay, and in these respects Liveing's masterpiece has never been equalled.

An essential part of Liveing's vision (and in this he was more related to Willis and Whytt than to his contemporaries) was the realization that the varieties of migraine were endless in number, and that they coalesced with many other paroxysmal reactions. His own theory of "nerve storms," of great generality and power, explained, as no other theory could, the sudden or gradual metamorphoses so characteristic of migraine attacks. The same thesis was expanded by Gowers, who portrayed migraine, faints, vagal attacks, vertigo, sleep disorders, and the like, as related to one another and to epilepsy—all such nerve-storms being mutually if mysteriously transformable amongst themselves.

The present century has been characterized both by advances and retrogressions in its approach to migraine. The advances reflect sophistications of technique and quantitation, and the retrogressions represent the splitting and fracturing of the subject which appears inseparable from the specialization of knowledge. By a historical irony, a real gain of knowledge and technical skill has been coupled with a real loss in general understanding.

A migraine is a physical event which may also be from the start, or later become, an emotional or symbolic event. A migraine expresses both physiological and emotional needs: it is the prototype of a psychophysiological reaction. Thus the convergence of thinking which its understanding demands must be based, simultaneously, both on neurology and on psychiatry (the convergence envisaged and brought nearer by Cannon, the physiologist, and Groddeck, the analyst); finally, migraine cannot be conceived as an exclusively human reaction, but must be considered as a form of biological reaction specifically tailored to human needs and human nervous systems.

The fragments of migraine must be gathered together and presented, once more, as a coherent whole. There have been innumerable technical papers and monographs which have extended and crystallized our knowledge of specific aspects of the subject. But there has not been a general essay since the time of Liveing.

Part I

The EXPERIENCE
of MIGRAINE

Oliver Sacks

partial [illegible] in always in the
individual — the individual's
experience of struggle [with]
something[?] [illegible] disorder

Introduction

Our first problem arises from the word *migraine*, which implies the existence of a (hemicranial) headache as a defining characteristic. It is necessary to state, at the very outset, that headache is *never* the sole symptom of a migraine, nor indeed is it a necessary feature of migraine attacks. We shall have occasion to consider many types of attack which exhibit every characteristic of migraines–clinically, physiologically, pharmacologically, and otherwise—but lack a headache component. We must retain the word *migraine* in view of its long and customary usage, but allow its extension far beyond the limits of any dictionary definition.

A variety of different syndromes may be recognized within the migraine syndrome, and these may overlap, merge, and metamorphose into one another. The most frequently occurring of these is the *common migraine* in which we find an assortment of migrainous symptoms grouped around the cardinal symptom of migraine headache (chapter 1). When components other than headache come to dominate an otherwise similar clinical picture, we may speak of *migraine equivalents*, and under this head we will consider periodic and recurrent attacks dominated by nausea and vomiting, abdominal pain, diarrhea, fever, drowsiness, mood changes, and the like (chapter 2). We must also discuss, in conjunction with these, certain other forms of attack and reaction which bear a clear if more remote relation to migraine: motion sickness, fainting, vagal attacks, and so on.

Separate consideration must be given to a peculiarly acute and dramatic type of attack—the *migraine aura*. Such auras may occur

11

as isolated events, or they may be followed by headache, nausea, and other features of the migraine complex. The entire syndrome, in the latter event, is termed a *classical migraine* (chapter 3).

Somewhat isolated from the above syndromes is a highly distinctive variant of migraine which has been described under a variety of names, and is best termed *migrainous neuralgia*. Very rarely, a common or classical migraine may be followed by long-lasting neurological deficits: these are termed *hemiplegic* or *ophthalmoplegic migraines*. In conjunction with these rare variants we will allude to *pseudo-migraines*, the mimicking of true migraines by organic lesions (chapter 4).

Part I concludes with an attempt to define, in the terms already employed, some formal characteristics common to all types of migraine attack, that is, the general structure of migraine.

1

Common Migraine

Since about my twentieth year, though otherwise in good health, I have suffered from migraine. Every three or four weeks I am liable to an attack. . . . I wake with a general feeling of disorder, and a slight pain in the region of the right temple which, without overstepping the mid-line, reaches its greatest intensity at midday; towards evening it usually passes off. While at rest the pain is bearable, but it is increased by motion to a high degree of violence. . . . It responds to each beat of the temporal artery. The latter feels, on the affected side, like a hard cord, while the left is in its normal condition. The countenance is pale and sunken, the right eye small and reddened. At the hight of the attack, when it is a violent one, there is nausea. . . . There may be left behind a slight gastric disorder; frequently, also, the scalp remains tender at one spot the following morning. . . . For a certain period after the attack I can expose myself with impunity to influences which before would have infallibly caused an attack.

—du Bois Reymond, 1860

The cardinal symptoms of common migraine are headache and nausea. Complementing these may be a remarkable variety of other major symptoms, in addition to minor disorders and physiological changes of which the patient may not be aware. Presiding over the entire attack there will be, in du Bois Reymond's words, "a general feeling of disorder," which may be experienced in either physical or emotional terms, and tax or elude the patient's powers of description. Great variability of symptoms is characteristic, not only of attacks in different patients, but between successive attacks in the same patient.

These, then, are the *ingredients* of a common migraine. We will list and describe them one by one, while understanding that migrainous symptoms never occur in such schematic isolation, but are linked to one another in various ways. Some symptoms are conjoined to form characteristic *constellations*, while others present themselves in a definite and often dramatic order, so that we may recognize a basic *sequence* to the attacks.

Headache

The *character* of the pains varied very much; most frequently they were of a hammering, throbbing or pushing nature . . . [in other cases] pressing and dull . . . boring with sense of bursting . . . pricking . . . rending . . . stretching . . . piercing . . . and radiating . . . in a few cases it felt as if a wedge was pressed into the head, or like an ulcer, or as if the brain was torn, or pressed outwards.

—Peters, 1853

Migraine headache is traditionally described as a violent throbbing pain in one temple, and not infrequently takes this form. It is impossible, however, to specify a constant site, quality, or intensity, for in the course of a specialized practice one will encounter all conceivable varieties of head pain in the context of migraine. Wolff, whose experience is unmatched in this area, has stated (1963):

The sites of the migraine headache are notably temporal, supra-orbital, frontal, retrobulbar, parietal, postauricular, and occipital. . . They may occur as well in the malar region, in the upper and the lower teeth, at the base of the nose, in the median wall of the orbit, in the neck and in the region of the common carotid arteries, and down as far as the tip of the shoulder.

One may say, however, that migraine headache is unilateral in *onset* more frequently than not, although it tends to become diffuse in distribution later in the attack. One side is generally attacked by preference, and in a few patients there may be an invariable left- or right-sided involvement throughout life. More commonly there is only a relative preference, often associated with the severity of pain: severe frequent hemicrania on one side with mild occasional hemicrania on the opposite side. A number of patients complain of an alternation of hemicrania from one side to the other in successive attacks, or even in the same attack. At least a third of all patients experience a bilateral or diffuse headache (holocrania) from the outset of the attack.

The *quality* of migraine headache is similarly variable. Throbbing occurs in less than half of all cases, and in these may characterize the headache only at its inception, soon giving way to a steady aching. Continued throbbing throughout the attack is uncommon, and occurs chiefly in those who drive themselves to continued physical activity despite a migraine. Throbbing, when it occurs, is synchronized with arterial pulsation, and may be accompanied by visible pulsation of extracranial arteries.

Its intensity is proportional to the increased amplitude of such arterial pulses (Wolff), and the pain may be interpreted by pressure on the affected artery, or the common carotid artery, or sometimes the eyeball, on the affected side. Such occlusion is immediately followed, when the finger is released, by a violent resurgence of the arterial pulse and the head pain. Throbbing is not, however, a *sine qua non* of vascular headache, and its absence does not have the significance of its occurrence. One may say, however, that almost all vascular headaches are aggravated by active or passive head-movement, by exertion or tension, or by the transmitted impulse of coughing, sneezing or vomiting. The pain is therefore minimized by rest, or by splinting of the head in one position. It may also be mollified by counter-pressure; many migraine sufferers will press the affected temple into their pillows, or hold the affected side with their hand.

The *duration* of migraine headache is extremely variable. In severely acute attacks (migrainous neuralgia), the pain may last only a matter of minutes. In a common migraine, the duration is rarely less than three hours, is commonly of eight to twenty-four hours' duration, and on occasion may last several days, or in excess of a week. Tissue changes may become manifest in very extended attacks. The superficial temporal artery (or arteries) may become exquisitely tender to the touch and visibly indurated. The surrounding skin may also become tender, and remain in this state for more than a day following the subsidence of the headache. Very rarely a spontaneous hygroma or hematoma may form about the affected vessel.

The *intensity* of migrainous headache is extremely variable. It may be of incapacitating violence, or so faint that its presence is only detected by the transient pain consequent upon jolting of the head or coughing.* Nor need the intensity remain constant throughout the attack; a slow waxing and waning with a period of a few minutes is commonly described, and much longer remissions and exacerbations may also occur, particularly in protracted menstrual migraines.

Migrainous headache is frequently complicated by the simultaneous or antecedent occurrence of other types of head pain. Characteristic "tension headache," localized especially in the cervical and posterior occipital regions, may inaugurate a migraine headache, or accompany it, particularly if the attack is marked by irritability, anxiety, or continued activity throughout its duration. Such tension-headache must not be construed as an integral portion of the migraine, but as a secondary reaction to it.

Nausea and Associated Symptoms

Eructations occur, either inodorous and without taste, or of an insupportable mawkishness; abundant mucosities and salivary fluid flow into the mouth, intermixed at times with those of a bitter, bilious taste; there is extreme disgust for food; general *malaise* . . . paroxysmal distensions of the stomach with gas, followed by belchings, with transient relief; or vomiting may occur. . . .

—Peters, 1853

Nausea is invariable in the course of a common migraine, whether it is trifling and intermittent, or continuous and overwhelming. The term *nausea* is used, and has always been used, in both literal and figurative senses, as denoting not only a specific (if unlocalizable) sensation, but a state of mind and pattern of behavior—a turning away, from food, from everything, and a turning inward. Even if there is no overt nausea, a vast majority of migraine patients will be averse to eating during the attack, knowing that the act of eating,

*The early literature provides some remarkable examples of "splitting" headaches. Thus Tissot (1790) records in his treatise: "C. Pison (a physician) experienced on himself such violent attacks of migraine that he believed his skull's sutures were splitting. . . . Stalpart Van der Viel *saw* the sutures of the skull actually splitting in an attack of migraine, the object of which was the gardener's wife . . ."

the sight, the smell, or even the very thought of food may bring on overwhelming nausea. We might almost speak of *latent* nausea in this connection.

A variety of other symptoms, local and systemic, are likely to be associated with nausea. Increased salivation and reflux of bitter stomach-contents (waterbrash), with the necessity of swallowing or spitting, may not only accompany the sensation of nausea, but precede it by several minutes. Not uncommonly, patients are alerted to the imminence of a severe sick-headache by finding their mouths filled with saliva or waterbrash, and may be enabled, by this timely signal, to take appropriate medication and ward off further oncoming symptoms.

Established nausea provokes various forms of visceral ejaculation; hiccup, belching, retching, and vomiting. If the patient is fortunate, vomiting may terminate not only his nausea but the entire migraine attack; more commonly, he will fail to secure relief from vomiting, and suffer instead an excruciating aggravation of concurrent vascular headache. When florid, nausea is far less tolerable than headache or other forms of pain, and in many patients, especially youthful ones, nausea and vomiting dominate the clinical picture and constitute the crowning misery of common migraine.

Repeated vomiting first empties the existing stomach-contents, is followed by vomiting of regurgitated bile, and finally by repeated "dry" heaving or retching. It is the chief cause (in company with profuse sweating and diarrhea) of the severe fluid and electrolyte depletion which can prostrate patients suffering protracted attacks.

Nausea is not only a physical symptom but a state-of-mind, a state-of-being, of a profoundly unpleasant and negative sort—the sort of existential state described in Sartre's "Nausea." For this reason it can cause a degree of misery, and an undermining of morale, beyond anything caused by headache or pain. It is nausea, above all, which can make one "sick of life," and cause that dire state described by Aretaeus two thousand years ago: "Life becomes a burden. . . . The patients are weary and wish to die."

Facial Appearance

The picturesque terms *red migraine* and *white migraine* were introduced by du Bois Reymond, and retain a certain descriptive value.

In a red migraine, the face is dusky and flushed: in the words of an old account:

congested, with rushing and roaring in the head, bloating, glowing, and shining of the face, with protrusion of the eyes . . . great heat of the head and face . . . throbbing of the carotid and temporal arteries . . .

—Peters, 1853

A full-blown, plethoric appearance, as Peters describes, is distinctly uncommon, occurring in less than a tenth of cases of common migraine. Patients predisposed to red migraines often have a marked propensity to flush with anger or blush with embarrassment: facial erythema, we may say, is their "style":

Case 40

A 60-year-old man of irascible temperament subject to common migraines since the age of 18, and bilious attacks and severe motion-sickness in childhood. He has a beef-red face, with tiny dilated arterioles in the nose and eyes. He flushes in his frequent rages, and indeed his face always seems to glow with a red smouldering fire which is the precise physiological counterpart of his chronic smouldering irritability. His face becomes crimson a few minutes before the onset of migraine headache, and remains flushed throughout the attack.

Much more familiar is the picture of white migraine, in which the face is pale, or even ashen, thin, drawn and haggard, while the eyes appear small, sunken, and ringed. These changes may be so marked as to suggest the picture of surgical shock. Intense pallor is always seen if there is severe nausea. On occasion, the face becomes flushed in the first few minutes of an attack, and then abruptly pale, as if, in Peters' words, "all the blood passed suddenly from the head to the legs."

Edema of the face and scalp may occur, either as isolated features or in the context of a very general fluid-retention and edema (see p. 23). Facial, lingual, and labial swelling, reminiscent of an angioneurotic edema, may occur at the inception of the attack in some patients. In one such patient whom I was able to observe at the inauguration of an attack, a massive periorbital edema developed on one side a few minutes before the onset of headache. More commonly, facial and scalp edema develop *after* prolonged dilatation of extracranial vessels, and are associated, as Wolff and others have shown, with fluid transudation and sterile inflammation about the involved vessels. The edematous skin is always tender and has a lowered pain-threshold.

Ocular Symptoms

It is almost always possible to detect changes in the appearance of the *eyes* during or before an attack of migraine headache, even though the patient himself may not volunteer any visual or ocular symptoms. There is usually some suffusion of small vessels in the globe, and in particularly severe attacks the eyes may become grossly bloodshot (this feature is characteristic in attacks of migrainous neuralgia). The eyes may appear moist (chemotic) from an increase in lacrimation—analogous to, and often synchronized with, the increased salivation—or bleary from an exudative inflammation of the vascular bed. Alternatively, the eyes may appear lusterless and sunken: a true enophthalmos may occur.

These changes in the eyeball, when severe, may be associated with a variety of symptoms: itching and burning in the affected eye(s), a painful sensitivity to light, and blurring of vision. Blurring of vision may be of incapacitating severity (blind-headache) and one may find it impossible to visualize the retinal vessels with any clarity at such times, due to the exudative thickening of the cornea.

Nasal Symptoms

Descriptions of migraine rarely pay much attention to nasal symptoms, although careful questioning of patients will reveal that at least a quarter of them develop some "stuffiness" of the nose in the course of an attack. Examination at this time will show engorged and purple turbinates. Such symptoms and findings, when they are present, may mislead both patient and physician into making a diagnosis of "sinus" or "allergic" headache.

Another nasal symptom, which may come either toward the beginning or at the resolution of the attack, is a profuse catarrhal secretion. It will be readily understandable that the combination of a running nose with a sense of malaise and headache may mimic a "cold" or other viral infection, and there can be no doubt but that a number of such migraines are misdiagnosed as such. When, however, the "cold" shows some propensity to occur every weekend, or after acute emotional disturbances, the true diagnosis may become apparent.

The following case history will illustrate how conspicuous a part may be played by nasal and other secretions in the course of a migraine, as well as certain other premonitory symptoms to be discussed later:

Case 20

A 53-year-old lady who has had common migraines of unusually elaborate format for nearly thirty years. At one time she used to have "a feeling of extreme well-being" the night before her attacks. More recently, she has tended to have feelings of intense drowsiness during the preceding evening, accompanied by repeated and uncontrollable yawning. She lays stress on the "unnatural . . . irresistible . . . ominous" qualities of this drowsiness. She will go to bed early, and her sleep will be of unusual length and density.

She will awake the next morning with what she terms "a feeling of unrest. . . . My whole system is set off in some way, and everything starts to move inside me. . . ." This feeling of unrest and internal motion resolves itself into a diffuse secretory activity, with profuse catarrh, salivation, lacrimation, sweating, water diuresis, vomiting, and diarrhea. After two or three hours of this massive internal activity she develops an intense throbbing headache on the left side.

Abdominal Symptoms and Abnormal Bowel Action

About one-tenth of adults who suffer from common migraine complain of abdominal pain or abnormal bowel action during the course of the attack. The proportion is notably higher in younger patients, and the abdominal symptoms described here as a minor component of a common migraine may constitute the predominant or only symptoms in so-called "abdominal migraines" (see chapter 2).

Two types of abdominal pain are described with some frequency: the first is an intense, steady, boring, "neuralgic" type of pain, usually felt in the upper abdomen and sometimes radiating to the back—it may mimic the pain of a perforated ulcer, cholecystitis, or pancreatitis. Somewhat more commonly, the patient describes a colicky abdominal pain, often referred to the right lower quadrant, and not infrequently taken for appendicitis.

Abdominal distension, visceral silence, and constipation tend to occur in the prodromal or earlier portions of a migraine, and contrast-studies performed at this stage have confirmed that there is stasis and dilation throughout the entire gastrointestinal tract. This is succeeded in the later or closing portions of the attack by increased peristaltic activity throughout the gut, clinically manifest as colicky pain, diarrhea, and gastric regurgitation.

Lethargy and Drowsiness

Although many patients, especially indomitable and obsessional ones, make no concessions to a migraine and insist on driving themselves through the usual round of work and play, a degree of listlessness and a desire for rest are characteristic of all severe common migraines. A vascular headache exquisitely sensitive to motion of the head may in itself enforce inactivity, but we cannot accept this as the only, or even the chief, mechanism at work. Many patients feel weak during an attack and exhibit diminished tone of skeletal muscles. Many are dejected, and seek seclusion and passivity. Many are drowsy.

The relation of sleep to migraine is a complex and fundamental one, and we will have occasion to touch upon it in many different contexts: the incidence of syncope and stupor in the acutest forms of migraine (migraine aura and classical migraine), the tendency for migraines of all types to occur during sleep, and their putative relation to dream and nightmare states. At this point we must pay attention to three aspects of a complex relationship: the occurrence of intense drowsiness or stupor before or during a common migraine, the occasional abortion of attacks by a short sleep of unusual density, and the typical protracted sleep in which many attacks find their natural termination.

Nowhere in the literature can we find more vivid and accurate descriptions of migrainous stupor than in Liveing's monograph.

It is important [he writes] to distinguish this drowsiness from the comparatively natural and graceful sleep which, in a large proportion of cases, terminates, and sometimes shortens the paroxysm. It is, on the contrary, of a most uncomfortable and oppressive character, sometimes verging on coma.

Liveing compares this drowsiness with the altered states of consciousness which may sometimes precede an asthmatic attack, citing the following introspective description of the latter:

Symptoms of an approaching fit began to appear at 4 p.m. The principal were fullness in the head, dullness and heaviness of the eyes, and disagreeable drowsiness. The drowsiness increased so much that I spent a great part of the evening in a succession of "trances," as I call them. This horrid drowsiness generally prevents one from being sensible of the approach of a fit till it has commenced.

I have already cited a case from my own experience (case 20,) in which the patient described a very similar state of irresistible and unpleasantly toned drowsiness as a prodromal feature of her attacks, and such descriptions may be multiplied manifold. Sometimes the drowsiness may precede other symptoms by minutes or hours, while at other times it presents itself *pari passu* with the headache and other symptoms. Repeated yawning is a characteristic feature of these lethargic states, presumably an attempted arousal mechanism to stave off the torpor. Migrainous drowsiness is not only "irresistible," glutinous and unpleasantly toned, but tends to be charged with peculiarly vivid, atrocious and incoherent dreams, a state verging on delirium. It is best, therefore, not to yield to it.*

Some patients do, however, discover that a brief deep sleep near the commencement of a migraine may prevent its subsequent evolution.

Case 18

A 24-year-old man who suffers both from classical and common migraines, and has experienced, on other occasions, both nocturnal asthmas and somnambulistic episodes. He finds that he may fall into a 'very deep sleep . . . they can hardly wake me' shortly after the onset of a migraine, and that if

---

*The "nightmare" song in *Iolanthe* provides a splendid description, not of a nightmare, but of a migraine delirium (the song mentions eleven other symptoms of migraine). As Gilbert and Sullivan observe: "Your slumbering teems with such horrible dreams that you'd much better be waking."

circumstances permit him to do this, he will awake within an hour with a sense of great refreshment, and the complete dispersal of all his symptoms. If he is prevented from sleeping in this fashion, the attack runs its course for the remainder of the day.

The duration of such curative sleeps may be very brief. Liveing cites the case of a gardener with typical abdominal migraines; this patient was able to abort the development of a full-blown attack if he could lie down under a tree and secure a ten minutes' sleep at its inception.

Dizziness, Vertigo, Faintness, and Syncope

True vertigo must be considered quite exceptional in the course of a common migraine, although it is often experienced in a migraine aura or classical migraine. Milder states of "light-headedness" occur with notable frequency. Selby and Lance (1960), in a clinical study of 500 patients with migraine of all types, found that "some 72 percent complained of a sensation of dizziness, lightheadedness and unsteadiness. . . . " They further observed that "sixty patients of 396 had lost consciousness in association with attacks of headache."

The possible causes of such symptoms may, of course, be multiple, and will include autonomic reactions to pain and nausea, vasomotor collapse, prostration due to fluid loss or exhaustion, muscular weakness and adynamia, and so on, in addition to the action of direct central mechanisms inhibiting the level of consciousness.

Alterations of Fluid Balance

A number of migraine patients complain of increased weight, or tightness of clothes, rings, belts, shoes, and so forth in association with their attacks. These symptoms have been submitted to precise experimental investigation by Wolff. Some weight gain preceded the headache stage in more than a third of the patients he studied; since however the headache could not be influenced either by experimental diuresis or hydration, Wolff concluded that "weight gain and widespread fluid retention are concomitant but not causally related to headache," an important conclusion which we shall have occasion to refer to when we come to discuss the interrelationship of different symptoms in the migraine complex.

During the period of water-retention urine is diminished in output and highly concentrated.* The retained fluid is discharged through a profuse diuresis, sometimes associated with other secretory activities, as the migraine attack resolves.

Case 35

This 24-year-old woman has invariable menstrual migraines and one or two further attacks in the course of an average month. Both menstrual and extramenstrual attacks are preceded by a weight-gain which may be as much as 10 lb; the fluid is distributed in the trunk, feet, hands, and face, and takes about two days to accumulate. Coincident with the fluid-retention is "a great increase in nervous energy," as the patient terms it, characterized by restlessness, hyperactivity, loquacity, and insomnia. This is followed by a 24- to 36-hour period of intestinal cramps and vascular headache. The detumescence of these attacks occurs, very literally, with a massive diuresis and an involuntary epiphora.

Fever

Many patients may complain that they *feel* feverish during the course of a common migraine, and they may indeed demonstrate flushing of the face, coldness and cyanosis of the extremities, shivering, sweating, and alternating feelings of heat and cold preceding or accompanying the onset of headache. These symptoms are not necessarily accompanied by fever, although the latter *may* be present, and are of considerable severity, especially in youthful patients.

Case 60

A 20-year-old man with a history of common migraines going back to his eighth year. The headaches are accompanied by intense nausea, pallor and

---

*I have had one patient, an intelligent woman whose testimony I am inclined to trust, who affirms that she develops a peculiar fruity odor in the periods of water-retention which inaugurate her occasional migraines. Unfortunately, however, she had no attacks during the six-month period that I saw her, so that no opportunity presented itself of identifying the nature or cause of this odor.

gastrointestinal disturbances, chills, cold sweats, and occasional rigors. I had the opportunity of examining him while he was in the throes of a severe attack, and found an oral temperature of 103.5°F.

Minor Symptoms and Signs

Contraction of one pupil, ptosis and enophthalmos (Horner's syndrome) may produce a striking asymmetry in cases of unilateral migraine. There is no consistency, however, concerning pupillary size. In the earlier stages of the attack, or if pain is very intense, the pupils may be enlarged; later in an attack, or if nausea, lethargy, collapse, and the like, dominate the picture, small pupils will be seen. The same considerations apply to pulse rate: an initial tachycardia is likely to be followed by a protracted bradycardia, the latter sometimes associated with significant hypotension and postural faintness or syncope. Observant patients may comment on such changes of pulse and pupil during their worst attacks.

Case 51

A 48-year-old man has had migraines since childhood, and also suffers from chronic tachycardia. He has been struck, therefore, by the slowing of his pulse during the attacks, and has also observed that his pupils, normally large, become minute. I was able to confirm these observations while seeing him in the course of an attack: there was striking pallor and diaphoresis, congested chemotic eyes, pinpoint pupils, and a bradycardia of 45.

There is no end to the number of odd, miscellaneous alterations of physiological function which *may* occur as a result of migraine; a complete listing of these would provide a fascinating catalogue of *curiosa*. It will suffice, however, to make brief reference to the occurrence of widespread vascular changes and occasional trophic changes associated with migraines. We have already noted that a spontaneous effusion or ecchymosis may develop about an involved scalp artery. I have had the opportunity of seeing one patient whose "red" migraines were associated with flushing of the entire body, followed, in the later portions of the attack, by the development of many spontaneous ecchymoses on the trunk and limbs. Another patient, a woman of 25, suffered pain in the palms of both hands with her migraine headaches; during the painful period the hands appeared flushed and congested: this syndrome is very similar to the "palmar migraine" described by Wolff.

The literature makes many references to whitening and loss of scalp hair following repeated migraines. The only case suggestive of this, in my own experience, was that of a middle-aged woman who had had very severe, frequent attacks of invariably left-sided hemicrania, and in her mid-twenties developed a startling streak of white hair on this side, the remainder of her hair remaining jet-black until many years later.

Organic Irritability

. . . the patient could not bear anything to touch his head, and the least sight or sound, even the ticking of his watch, was insupportable.
—Tissot, 1778

Irritability and photophobia are exceedingly common in the course of migraine attacks, and have been adopted, by Wolff and others, as pathognomonic features aiding the diagnosis.

We are concerned with two types of irritability as accompaniments of the migraine state. The first is an aspect of the mood change and defensive seclusion which may be so prominent in the behavior and social posture of many migraine patients. The second type of irritability arises from a diffuse sensory excitation and excitability so great that it may render all sensory stimuli intolerable, as the old words of Tissot remind us. In particular, migraine patients are prone to photophobia, an intense discomfort, both local and general, provoked by light, and an avoidance of light which may become the most obvious external characteristic of the entire attack. Some of this photophobia is on the basis of conjunctival hyperemia and inflammation, as described earlier, and is associated with burning and smarting of the eyes. But a major component of photophobia is a central irritability and sensory arousal, which may be accompanied by very vivid and protracted visual after-images and turbulent visual imagery. Alvarez has provided a graphic description of such symptoms in himself; during the early part of his own migraines, he sees such brilliant after-images on his television screen that he is unable to watch the picture. Observant patients frequently note, if they close their eyes at such a time, that they are submitted to an involuntary visual barrage, a kaleidoscope presentation of rapidly changing colors and images, the latter either crude or as highly organized as dream images.

An exaggeration and intolerance of sound—phonophobia—is equally characteristic of the severe attack; distant sounds, the noise of traffic, or the dripping of a tap, may appear unbearably loud and provoke the patient to fury.

Very characteristic of this state is an exaggeration, and often a perversion of the sense of smell; delicate perfumes appear to stink, and may elicit an overwhelming reaction of nausea. Similarly with the sense of taste, the blandest foods acquiring intense and often disgusting flavors.

It is important to note that sensory excitability of this type may precede the onset of headache, and, in general, is characteristic of the *early* portions of the migraine attack. It is often followed by a state of sensory inhibition or indifference for the remainder of the attack: in Peters' words, "by general hebetude of sensorial power . . . " The alterations of sensation and sensory threshold which occur in common migraine, however distressing to the patient, are very mild in comparison to the intense hallucinations and perversions of sensation which are characteristic of migraine aura and classical migraine.

Mood Changes

The interrelationship of affective states and migraine is one of the greatest complexity, and as such will demand repeated exploration as we traverse the subject. Obvious difficulties present themselves, from the start, in distinguishing cause and effect, and very careful questioning, or observation over a prolonged period, may be needed to dissect out those affective changes which form an *integral* part of the migraine syndrome from antecedent moods and feelings which have played a part in precipitating the attack, and from the secondary, emotional consequences of the attack itself.

When these factors have been duly weighed, we will continue to be struck by the fact that profound affective changes may occur during, and only during, a migraine attack, changes which are particularly startling in patients of normally equable temperament. Moreover, it will become clear that such mood changes are not simply reactions to pain, nausea, and other occurrences, but are themselves primary symptoms proceeding *concurrently* with the many other symptoms of the attack. Very profound mood changes may also occur *before* and *after* the bulk of the attack, and as such will be considered in the concluding section of this chapter. The most important emotional colorings during the clinically recognized portion of a common migraine are states of anxious and irritable hyperactivity in the early portions of the attack, and states of apathy and depression in the bulk of the attack.

The common picture of anxious irritability has already been sketched in the preceding section. The patient is restless and agitated; if confined to his bed, he will move about constantly, rearranging the bedclothes, finding no position of comfort; he will tolerate neither sensory nor social intrusions. His irascibility may be extreme. Such states are exacerbated if the patient continues to drive himself through his habitual routine of work, and their exacerbation, by a vicious circle, is likely to provoke a further increase in other symptoms of the attack.

Very different is the picture presented in the fully established or protracted attack. Here the physical and emotional posture is characterized by accepting suffering, dejection and passivity. Such patients, unless compelled to act otherwise by internal or external factors, *withdraw* or regress into illness, solitude and seclusion. The emotional depression at such times is very real, often serious, and occasionally suicidal. The following account is taken from an eighteenth-century description:

From the first perception of uneasiness in the stomach the spirits begin to flag. They grow more and more depressed, until cheerful thoughts and feelings fly away, and the patient conceives himself the most wretched of human beings and feels as if he were never to be otherwise. . . .

This old description brings out the true depressive quality—the sense of utter hopelessness and permanence of misery—a reaction which is clearly far in excess of a realistic response to a short-lived benign attack of which the patient has had innumerable experiences.

Feelings of depression will be associated with feelings of anger and resentment, and in the severest migraines there may exist a very ugly mixture of despair, fury and loathing of everything and everyone, not excluding the self. Such states of enraged helplessness may be intolerable both for the patient and his family, and their potential severity must never be underrated by the physician who undertakes to look after the severely incapacitated and depressed patient in the throes of an attack.

Symptom-Constellations in Common Migraine

We have now listed the major symptoms of a common migraine *as if* they were unrelated to one another and occurred at random. Certain groups of symptoms tend, however, to occur with some consistency. Thus, severe vascular headache usually occurs in association with the other evidences of dilatation in extracranial vessels: suffusion and chemosis of the eyes, vascular engorgement within the nose, facial flushing, and so on. In other patients, gastrointestinal symptoms form a coherent phalanx: gastric and intestinal distension, abdominal pains, followed by diarrhea and vomiting. A "shock" picture is seen in severe "white" migraines, constituted by pallor, coldness of the extremities, profuse cold sweating, chilliness, shivering, slowness and feebleness of the pulse, and postural hypotension; this picture is frequently seen in association with very severe nausea, but many occur when nausea is not prominent. In such constellations, there is a fairly obvious physiological linkage of the symptoms, an expected concurrence. The type of conjunction is less readily explained in certain other constellations which tend to occur, in particular, in the earliest or prodromal stages of the attack, or during its resolution. Thus we may recognize, in the former case, a tendency for hunger, thirst, constipation, physical and emotional hyperactivity to be linked together; or, in the latter case, for a great number of secretory activities to proceed in unison.

The Sequence of a Common Migraine

A migraine attack is likely to be described by the patient in terms of a single symptom, or a mass of symptoms. Patient questioning and observation of repeated attacks may be necessary before it becomes clear that there is a preferred order or sequence of symptoms. The appreciation of such a sequence at once raises problems of terminology and definition: What constitutes the attack "proper"? Where does it begin and end?

As generally understood and described, a common migraine is constituted by vascular headache, nausea, increased splanchnic activity (vomiting, diarrhea, etc.), increased glandular activity (salivation, lacrimation, etc.), muscular weakness and atonia, drowsiness and depression. We will find, however, that migraine neither starts nor ends with these symptoms, but is both preceded and followed by symptoms and states which are clinically and physiologically the reverse of these.

We may speak of premonitory or *prodromal symptoms*, while recognizing that these pass, insensibly, into the earlier phases of the attack proper. Some of these prodromal or early symptoms are local, some systemic; some are physical, and others are emotional. Among the more common physical prodromes we must include states of water-retention and thirst, states of visceral dilatation and constipation, states of muscular tension and sometimes hypertension. Among the emotional or psychophysical prodromes we must recognize states of hunger, restless hyperactivity, insomnia, vigilance, and emotional arousal which may have either an anxious or euphoric coloring. Thus George Eliot, herself a sufferer from severe common migraines, would speak of feeling "dangerously well" the day before her attacks. Such states, when they are acute and extreme, may achieve an almost maniacal intensity.

Case 63

This middle-aged man was of normally phlegmatic nature, and presented a forbidding austerity of appearance and manner. He had experienced infrequent common migraines since childhood, and described the prodromal excitement of these attacks with some embarrassment. For two or three hours before the onset of his headaches he would be "transformed": he would feel thoughts rushing through his head, and would have an almost uncontrollable tendency to laugh or sing or whistle or dance.

States of premigrainous excitement are more commonly of unpleasant tone, and take the form of irritable or agitated anxiety-states.

Very occasionally such states will reach panic or psychotic intensity. Affective prodromes of this type are particularly common as part of a premenstrual syndrome.

Case 71

A 29-year-old woman with stormy menstrual syndromes of great severity. The pre-menstrual phase would be marked by increasing water-retention for two days, accompanied by a crescendo of diffuse anxiety and irritability. Her sleep would be poor and punctuated by nightmares. The emotional disturbance would reach its maximum in the hours immediately preceding the menses, at which time the patient would become hysterical, violent, and hallucinated. The emotional state would return to normal within a few hours of the onset of menstruation, and be followed, the next day, by severe vascular headache and intestinal colic.

The *resolution* of a common migraine, or indeed of any variety of migraine attack, may proceed in three ways, as has been recognized since the seventeenth century. It may, in its natural course, exhaust itself and end in sleep; the postmigrainous sleep is long, deep, and refreshing, like a postepileptic sleep. Secondly, it may resolve by "lysis", a gradual abatement of the suffering accompanied by one or more secretory activities. As Calmeil wrote, almost 150 years ago:

Vomiting sometimes terminates a migraine. An abundant flow of tears does the same, or an abundant secretion of urine. Sometimes hemicrania is terminated by an abundant perspiration from the feet, hands, half of the face, or by a nose-bleeding, a spontaneous arterial hemorrhage, or a mucous flux from the nose.

One must, of course, add to Calmeil's list that an abundant diarrhea, or menstrual flow, may similarly accompany the resolution of a migraine. The hateful mood of a migraine—depressed and withdrawn, or furious and irascible—tends to melt away in the stage of lysis, to melt away *with* the physiological secretion. "Resolution by secretion" thus resembles a catharsis on both physiological and psychological levels, like weeping for grief. The following case history illustrates a number of these points.

Case 68

This 32-year-old man was an ambitious and creative mathematician whose life was geared to a weekly psychophysiological cycle. Toward the end of the working week, he would become fretful, irritable, and distractable, "useless" at anything save the simplest routine tasks. He would have difficulty sleeping on Friday nights, and on Saturdays would be unbearable. On Sunday mornings he would awaken with a violent migraine, and would be forced to remain in bed for the greater part of the day. Toward evening he would break out in a gentle sweat and pass many pints of pale urine. The fury of his sufferings would melt away with the passage of these secretions. Following the attack he would feel a profound refreshment, a tranquillity, and a surge of creative energy which would carry him to the middle of the following week.

The third mode of resolution of a migraine is by *crisis*—a sudden accession of physical or mental activity, which brings the attack to an end within minutes.

Violent physical exercise may avert an attack, or truncate an existing attack. Many patients who lie abed late on Sunday and wake with a migraine find that early rising and hard physical work will prevent its occurrence. One patient of mine, a mesomorphic Italian of a violent temperament, employs coitus to terminate his migraines if he is at home, or arm-wrestling if an attack comes on when he is at work, or drinking with his mates. Both are effective within five to ten minutes. Sudden fright, or rage, or other strong emotion may disperse and displace a migraine almost within seconds. One patient, asked how he terminated his attacks, said: "I have to get my adrenalin up. . . . I have got to run around, or shout, or get in a fight, and the headache vanishes." Various forms of paroxysmal visceral activity may accomplish the same end. Violent vomiting is the classical example, but other activities may be equally effective.

Case 66

This patient, whose migraines were invariably terminated by paroxysmal vomiting, developed an ulcer in middle life, and was submitted to subtotal gastrectomy and vagotomy. When he had his first migraine after the operation he found himself unable to vomit, and felt disconsolate. Suddenly, however, he started sneezing with extraordinary violence and when the fit of sneezing had subsided his migraine was gone. Subsequently he adopted the use of snuff to facilitate the resolution of his attacks, and in doing so has unwittingly adopted an eighteenth-century prescription.

Other patients may hiccup, or belch repeatedly, with rapid resolution of their attacks. Even voracious eating may secure an early abortion of the attack, monstrous as such an activity would appear to most migraine patients. The relief comes *with the act* of eating.*
Whichever method is utilized—violent physical, visceral, or emotional activity—the common factor is *arousal*. The patient is, as it were, awoken from his migraine as if from sleep. We shall further have occasion to see, when the specific drug therapies of migraine are under discussion, that the majority of these too serve to arouse the organism from a state of physiological depression.

We have already intimated an analogy between migraine and sleep, and this analogy is dramatized by the sense of extreme refreshment, and almost of rebirth, which may follow a severe but compact attack (see case 68). Such states do not represent a mere restoration to the premigraine condition, but a swing in the direction of arousal, a *rebound* after the migrainous trough. In the words of Liveing: "[the patient] awakes a different being." Rebound euphoria and refreshment is particularly common after severe menstrual migraines. It is least in evidence after a protracted attack with vomiting, diarrhea and fluid loss; such attacks fail to "recharge" the patient, and necessitate a period of convalescence.

One may describe an epilepsy simply in terms of the convulsion, while conceding that this may be preceded, in many patients, by a period of pre-ictal excitement and myoclonus, and followed by post-ictal stupor and exhaustion. But the violence and acuteness of the paroxysm justifies a restriction of the word *epilepsy* to cover this alone. In the case of a much more protracted paroxysmal reaction, like a migraine, it does not make sense—clinically, physiologically, or semantically—to limit the meaning of the word to the headache stage, or to any stage. The *entire sequence*—which we may then subdivide into prodromal stages, "attack proper," resolution, and rebound—must be denoted by the term *migraine*. If this is not done, it becomes impossible to comprehend the nature of migraine.

---

*Pavlov remarked on the frequency with which a hypnoidal state in a dog might be broken up by eating. The act of eating, often followed by scratching and sneezing, serves to arouse the dog from its trance-like state and was therefore termed by Pavlov an "autocurative" reflex.

In the attempt to clarify, one may oversimplify. I may not have emphasized, sufficiently, a rather characteristic, yet indefinable, state that is best called "unsettled." In this unsettled state, one may feel hot or cold or both; bloated and tight, or loose and queasy; a peculiar tension, a languor, or both; there are head pains, or other pains, sundry strains and discomforts, which come and go. *Everything* comes and goes, nothing is settled, and if one could take a total thermogram, or scan, or inner photograph of the body, one would see vascular beds opening and closing, peristalsis accelerating or stopping, viscera squirming or tightening in spasm, secretions suddenly increasing or lessening—*as if the nervous system itself was in a state of indecision*.

A medical friend of mine calls this "the autonomic jitters," a good term, for it evokes not only the autonomic instability but also the nervy, jittery state that goes along with this. At such times one may feel not only acutely ill but suffer a peculiar agitation and disquietude of mind, that *double* distress, of which Aretaeus speaks, which is at once, and inseparably, of Body and Mind.

After minutes or hours this unsettledness starts to "settle," but not into health, not alas ! into health, but into the fixed and settled forms of illness, those transfixed forms which are the "textbook" symptoms and signs of migraine.

McKenzie once called Parkinsonism "an organized chaos," and this is equally true of Migraine. First there is chaos, then organization, a sick order; it is difficult to know which is worse! The nastiness of the first lies in its uncertainty, its flux; the nastiness of the second in its sense of immutable heavy permanence. Typically, indeed, treatment is only possible early, before the migraine has "solidified" into immovable fixed forms.

2

Migraine Equivalents

Consideration of the many symptoms which may compose a common migraine has shown us that the term cannot be identified with any one symptom. A migraine is an aggregate of innumerable components, and its structure is composite. The emphasis of the components is extremely variable within the framework of a general pattern. Headache may be the cardinal symptom; it may constitute only a subsidiary symptom; it may even be entirely absent. We use the term *migraine equivalent* to denote symptom complexes which possess the generic features of migraine, but lack a specific headache component.

This term is comparable to that of "epileptic equivalent," which denotes a form of epilepsy without convulsion. We justify the use of the term "*migraine equivalent*" if the following circumstances are fulfilled: the occurrence of discrete noncephalgic attacks with a duration, a periodicity, and a clinical format similar to attacks of common migraine, and a tendency to be precipitated by the same type of emotional and physical antecedents. These clinical affinities will be matched, and confirmed, by physiological and pharmacological similarities.

Although earlier writers provided vivid case histories of different types of migraines ("gastric megrim," "visual megrim," etc.), it remained for Liveing to trace the mutual convertibility of such attacks, and to speak of "transformations" and "metamorphoses" in this context. Thus, he would speak of asthmatic, epileptic, vertiginous, gastralgic, pectoralgic, laryngismal, and maniacal "transformations" of migraine.

The notion of migraine equivalents has not, for the most part, been sympathetically received. The physician who presumes to diagnose an "abdominal migraine" will be regarded, by many of his colleagues, as talking mumbo-jumbo or worse, and it may only be after endless diagnostic investigations and negative laparotomies, or the sudden replacement of attacks of abdominal pain by typical vascular headaches, that the old Victorian term is exhumed and reconsidered.

The concentrated experience of working with migraine patients must convince the physician, whatever his previous beliefs, that many patients *do* suffer repeated, separate paroxysmal attacks of abdominal pain, chest pain, fever, and so forth, which fulfill every clinical criterion of migraine save for the presence of headaches. We will confine ourselves at this stage to a discussion of the following syndromes: cyclic vomiting and "bilious attacks," "abdominal migraines," "precordial migraines," and periodic, neurogenic disorders of body temperature, mood, and level of consciousness.

In addition to these acute, periodic, paroxysmal syndromes, there are a great variety of other states which bear *some* affinity to migraines, for example, "hangovers," reserpine reactions, and so forth. Consideration of these syndromes will be deferred to Part II.

Cyclic Vomiting and Bilious Attacks

We have observed the frequency and severity of nausea as a component of juvenile migraines. Frequently, it forms the cardinal symptom of a migraine reaction, and as such is often dignified with the term *bilious attack*. Selby and Lance provide the following figures from their large series:

. . . of 198 cases [of migraine] 31 percent recalled frequently occurring bilious attacks. Of a further 139 patients, 59 percent have a history of some bilious attacks or severe motion-sickness during their early years.

I have not tabulated incidence-figures from my own practice, but would estimate—in accordance with Selby and Lance's figures—that nearly half the migraine patients one questions have suffered such symptoms at one time or another. Severe nausea is always accompanied by multiple autonomic symptoms—pallor, shivering, diaphoresis, and the like. A majority of attacks are put down to dietary indiscretion in childhood, and in adult life ascribed to "gastric flu" or gall-bladder pathology, according to the persuasion of the physician.

Such attacks may persist throughout life, or may undergo a gradual or sudden transition to the "adult" form—common migraine. The following case history, provided by Vahlquist and Hackzell (1949), illustrates the genesis and evolution of such attacks in a young patient:

. . . When he was 10 months old he was badly frightened by an air-raid siren, and after this had abnormal fear-reactions and *pavor nocturnus*. . . . The first typical attack occurred at the age of one year. He suddenly turned pale, and later had an attack of violent vomiting. During the next two years he had several attacks a week, always of the same type. . . . When he was about three, he began to complain of a pain in his head during the attacks. . . . They generally ended in a heavy sleep.

We may note, in passing, that cyclic vomiting of this type is also commonly associated with abnormal rage reactions, and frequently coexists with temper tantrums.

Abdominal Migraine

The symptoms in any type of migraine are multiple, and the division between "bilious attacks" and "abdominal migraines" is an arbitrary one. The dominant feature in the latter is epigastric pain of continuous character and great severity, accompanied by a variety of further autonomic symptoms. The following incisive description is provided in Liveing's monograph:

When about 16 years old, enjoying otherwise excellent health, I began to suffer from periodic attacks of severe pain in the stomach. . . . The seizure would commence at any hour, and I was never able to discover any cause for it, for it was preceded by no dyspeptic symptoms or disordered bowels. . . . The pain began with a deep, ill-defined uneasiness in the epigastrium. This steadily increased in intensity during the next two or three hours, and then declined. When at its height the pain was very intolerable and sickening—it had no griping quality whatever. It was always accompanied by chilliness, cold extremities, a remarkably slow pulse, and a sense of nausea. . . . When the pain began to decline there was generally a feeling of movement in the bowels. . . . The paroxysm left very considerable tenderness of the affected region, which took a day or two to clear off, but there was no tenderness at the time.

Some years later, this particular patient ceased to have his abdominal attacks, but developed instead attacks of classical migraine coming at similar intervals of three to four weeks.

I have notes of more than forty patients (out of a total of 1,200) who consulted me with the presenting symptoms of common or classical migraine, but admitted to having had abdominal attacks similar to those described for months or years in the past. Observant patients may comment on the slowness of the pulse and other autonomic symptoms accompanying the abdominal pain. Thus a patient cited earlier (case 51) had for a period of five years abdominal attacks in place of his common migraines, but had observed slowing of the pulse, smallness of the pupils, suffusing of the eyes, and pallor in both types of attack. I have been given descriptions by three patients of what might be termed classical abdominal migraines.

Case 10

This 32-year-old man had suffered from classical migraines since the age of 10, the attacks coming with great regularity every four weeks. On some occasions, the migraine scotoma would be followed, not by headache, but by severe abdominal pain and nausea lasting six to ten hours.

An excellent account of the presentations of abdominal migraine in children, and the problems of diagnosis to which they may give rise, has been provided by Farquhar (1956).

Periodic Diarrhea

We have observed the frequency of diarrhea as a symptom in common migraine, especially in the later phases of the attack. Diarrhea per se, often preceded by severe constipation, may be abstracted as an isolated symptom occurring in the same circumstances, or with the same periodicity, as attacks of common migraine—one of the commonest of such complaints is "weekend diarrhea." Such neurogenic diarrheas tend to be ascribed to dietary indiscretion, or food-poisoning, or "intestinal flu," and so forth, until such explanations lose their acceptability, and it is borne in upon patient and physician that the attack represents a cyclic or circumstantial equivalent of migraine.

A certain number of such patients, especially those under severe chronic emotional stress, may proceed from a benign pattern of isolated migrainous diarrheas to a chronic mucous diarrhea, or, rarely, a true ulcerative colitis. One suspects, in such patients, that the bowel has been a "target organ" from the start.

Periodic Fever

High fever may occur in the course of severe common migraines, particularly in children. It may also be abstracted as an isolated periodic symptom occurring in its own right, and sometimes alternating with common migraines.

I have seen half a dozen patients, currently suffering from common or classical migraines, who have had such attacks of periodic neurogenic fever in the past. The differential diagnosis may be laborious and tricky in such cases, for all possible causes of organic disease must be considered and excluded before one dare postulate a functional or neurogenic origin for such a symptom. The following case history is summarized from Wolff:

The patient, an engineer aged 43, began suffering from intermittent attacks of fever up to 104° F in 1928, and he had continued to be afflicted with them . . . until 1940. It is of special interest that similar intermittent attacks of fever associated with "sick-headache," nausea and vomiting, had occurred in the patient's father. . . .

During late adolescence the patient himself began suffering from periodic headaches . . . especially frequent at times of emotional strain, and diagnosed as migraine. . . . Before each [febrile] episode there were prodromal symptoms . . . a feeling of unrest and difficulty in concentration. The temperature rose rapidly to a peak and returned to normal within twelve hours. Leucocytosis (in the neighborhood of 15,000 cells) occurred. After the fevers he had a "purged" feeling with a sense of especial well-being and mental efficiency.

This admirable case history illustrates that attacks of febrile migraine equivalent may present a similar sequence to attacks of common migraine, with prodromal "arousal," and postmigrainous rebound and replenishment. It may also be noted that the patient's fevers ceased following therapeutic discussion of his emotional problems and general situation, and the presumed mechanism of his attacks.

Precordial Migraine

The term *precordial migraine* (pectoralgic, or pseudoanginal migraine) denotes the occurrence of chest pain as a major constituent of a common or classical migraine, or its occurrence as a periodic, paroxysmal symptom with migrainous rather than anginal qualities and antecedents.

The symptom is a rare one, and I have encountered it only twice in my experience of over 1,000 migraine patients, once associated with common, and once with classical, migraines. The following case history illustrates its occurrence during, and alternating with, classical attacks:

Case 58

A 61-year-old woman who had had attacks of classical migraine since adolescence. The majority of her attacks are ushered in by scintillation and paraesthesiae, bilaterally, followed by intense unilateral vascular headache, nausea, and abdominal pain. A further symptom, during such severe attacks, is a feeling of painful tightness in the chest, accompanied by the radiation of pain to the left scapula, and down the left arm: it generally lasts for two to three hours.

The chest-pain is not aggravated by exercise, nor is it accompanied by cardiographic abnormalities; it is not alleviated by nitroglycerin, but is diminished, in company with its other accompanying symptoms, by ergotamine.

On occasion, this patient has had attacks of similar chest-pain occurring as an isolated symptom, and sometimes ushered in by migrainous scotomata and paraesthesiae.

The presentation and diagnosis of such attacks has been very fully considered by Fitz-Hugh (1940).

Periodic Sleep and Trance-States

The drowsiness which often accompanies or precedes a severe common migraine is occasionally abstracted as a symptom in its own right, and may then constitute the sole expression of the migrainous tendency. The following case illustrates the "transformation" of common migraine to a sleep equivalent.

Case 76

The patient was a nun who had been subject to common migraines of great severity at least twice weekly for some twenty years. Treatment was initially prophylactic and symptomatic in view of her wish to avoid discussion of personal matters. After three months of such treatment, her cephalgic attacks abruptly disappeared, but there occurred, in their stead, once or twice weekly sleeps of almost stuporous intensity. These attacks would last ten to fifteen hours, and constituted an unprecedented *addition* to her usual nocturnal sleep.

We have alluded to the frequency of torpor in postprandial migraines. The following case history, which we will have occasion to refer to in other contexts, illustrates the occurrence of postprandial stupors as an isolated symptom.

Case 49

The patient, an obsessively hard-working engineer—in his own words, "I never stop—I wish I didn't have to sleep"—suffers from a remarkable variety of migrainous equivalents and analogues. Unless he forces himself to take a brisk walk after meals, he will fall into an irresistible torpor. He describes this as follows: "I go into a trance, where I am able to hear things around me, but can't move. I am soaked with a cold sweat. My pulse gets very slow." The state lasts between one and two hours, rarely less or more than this. He "wakes," if one may use the word, with a feeling of intense refreshment and bounding energy.

We may also note briefly, at this stage, that migrainous sleeps and stupors not infrequently alternate with other and briefer periodic trance-states, such as narcolepsies, "daymares," and somnambulistic episodes. Particular attention will be paid to such relationships in later chapters.

Periodic Mood Changes

We have already spoken of the affective concomitants of common migraines—elated and irritable prodromal states, states of dread and depression associated with the main phase of the attack, and states of euphoric rebound. Any or all of these may be abstracted as isolated periodic symptoms of relatively short duration—some hours, or at most two or three days, and as such may present themselves as primary emotional disorders. The most acute of these mood changes, generally no more than an hour in duration, usually represents concomitants or equivalents of migraine aura. We may confine our attention at this stage to attacks of depression, or truncated manic-depressive cycles, occurring at intervals in patients who have previously suffered from attacks of undoubted (classical, common, abdominal, etc.) migraine. Alvarez, who is particularly alert to the occurrence of such migrainous equivalents, cites the following history:

A woman aged 56 complained of spells of deep depression lasting for a day or two. Her home physician thought they were probably menopausal in origin, but I found they were migrainous, and associated with a slight unilateral headache. I learned that in her early girlhood she had had spells of typically migrainous vomiting. . . . In her forties, she had had severe migrainous headaches with much retching.

An unusually clear-cut case from my own experience was provided by the following patient, part of whose history has already been cited in another context:

Case 10

This 32-year-old man had suffered both from classical cephalgic and classical abdominal migraines since childhood, the attacks coming with considerable regularity at monthly intervals. In his mid-twenties, he had been free of such attacks for more than a year, but suffered during this time from equally regular attacks of elation followed by severe depression, the entire episode lasting no more than two days.

Characteristic of such affective equivalents is their *brevity*—manic-depressive cycles, as generally understood, occupy several weeks, and frequently longer. Monthly affective equivalents of this type—or "lunacies" if we may venture the term—are most commonly seen in the context of menstrual syndromes.

Menstrual Syndromes

A large minority of women experience marked affective and autonomic disturbances about the time of menstruation. Greene has estimated that "about twenty women in every hundred suffer sometimes from premenstrual migraine," and if we include under this heading autonomic and affective disturbances not accompanied by headache, the figure must be substantially higher than this. Indeed, we may say that the menstrual cycle is *always* associated with some degree of physiological disturbance, even though this may pass unobserved by the patient. The disturbance tends to be in the direction of psychophysiological arousal prior to the menses, and "let-down" followed by rebound after the menses.

The arousal period may be characterized by "tension," anxiety, hyperactivity, insomnia, fluid-retention, thirst, constipation, abdominal distension, and so forth, and, more rarely, asthma, psychosis, or epilepsy. The "let-down" period, or "de-rousal," may be manifest as lassitude, depression, vascular headache, visceral hyperactivity, pallor, sweating, and the like. In short, virtually all symptoms of migraine, as they have been described thus far, may also be condensed into the biological turmoil surrounding menstruation.

Of particular relevance in the present context is the frequent alternation, during the life-history of a single patient, of differing formats of menstrual syndrome, with the emphasis on vascular headache at one time, at another on intestinal cramping, and so on. The following case history illustrates a sudden "transformation" between two types of menstrual migraine.

Case 32

A 37-year-old woman had experienced severe abdominal (probably intestinal) cramping at the menstrual period between the ages of 17 and 30. She suddenly ceased to experience these symptoms at that age, but suffered, in their place, typical premenstrual migraine headaches.

Other patients may suffer severe menstrual symptoms for several years, lose these to acquire frequent attacks of paroxysmal headache or abdominal pain unrelated to the menstrual periods, finally reverting to the original pattern of menstrual disturbance.

The precise timing of such menstrual syndromes, and their physiological and psychological relationship to menstruation, will be considered at length in chapter 8.

Alternations and Transformations

It is legitimate to speak of abdominal, precordial, febrile, affective, and the like, "equivalents" of migraine, in that the general format and sequence of migraine, as pictured in chapter 1, persists despite the varying emphasis of individual symptoms. There are, in addition to such acceptable equivalents, many other forms of paroxysmal illness or reaction which may insidiously or suddenly "replace" migraine attacks in the life-history of an individual; they occur, for the most part, with the same periodicity as the original migraines, or in response to much the same circumstances. It would be absurd, without doubt, to speak of paroxysmal asthma, angina, or laryngospasm as being migraine equivalents, yet clinical observation forces us to wonder whether they may not, on occasion, fill a biological role analogous to that of migraine attacks. Semantic argument is profitless in this context, and we may content ourselves, for the moment, with the noncommittal term which Liveing uses: *allied disorders*.

Heberden (1802) recorded the already established observation that "the hemicrania . . . has ceased upon the coming of an asthma," and it is impossible to doubt that there may be sudden transitions from one species of paroxysm to the other during the life-history of a patient. I have myself observed such alternations, generally abrupt, in at least twenty patients under my care. The following case history, already presented in part, typifies such a transformation.

Case 18

This 24-year-old man suffered from frequent nightmares and somnambulistic episodes until the age of 8, attacks of periodic, usually nocturnal, asthma until the age of 13, and classical and common migraines thereafter.

The classical migraines would come, with considerable regularity, every Sunday afternoon. The use of ergot compounds effectively aborted these attacks, and after three months of therapeutic care, he suddenly ceased to experience even the premonitory migraine auras. Some weeks after this he returned to me angrily complaining that his long-defunct attacks of asthma had returned, and that they came, in particular, on Sunday afternoons. He regretted the change, finding his migraines preferable to, and altogether less frightening than, the asthmas. "Give me back my migraine," he said.

We will have occasion to return to this particular and illuminating case history in the following chapter. This was one of my first patients, and his experience, our joint experience, early persuaded me that merely symptomatic treatment in certain patients might do no more than drive them through an endless repertoire of "allied reactions."

Similar case histories may be collected, and similar considerations adduced, with regard to the mutual transformations of migraine with attacks of neurogenic angina or laryngospasm, the former of these transformations also being well known to Heberden: "Instances are not wanting," he writes, " . . . where attacks of this complaint and now of headache have afflicted the patient by turns." Perplexing problems of differential diagnosis are presented by certain patients in whom attacks of *angina sine dolore*, neither precipitated by exercise nor accompanied by cardiographic changes alternate with migraines. The following description, taken from Beaumont (1952), shows the common clinical ground which may be shared by the two types of attack.

The patient is suddenly seized by a sensation of imminent death, becomes pale and motionless, and yet experiences no pain. During an attack salivation or vomiting may occur, the attack ceasing with eructation of wind, or a copious flow of urine.

Neurogenic laryngospasm (croup) provides another example of an exceptionally acute paroxysmal reaction which may show mutual transformations with attacks of migraine. An excellent example of this is provided by Liveing. We have already alluded to the abdominal migraines experienced by his patient "Mr. A" (periodic attacks between the ages of 16 and 19), and the attacks of classical migraine which succeeded these (between the ages of 19 and 37).

Subsequently, this patient "lost" his classical migraines, but suffered from periodic attacks of paroxysmal croup:

. . . after having been asleep an hour or so, he would suddenly wake to consciousness in the act of jumping out of bed, tearing open his collar-band and struggling violently for breath with loud stridulous breathing; after a few minutes of this, which appeared to him a prolonged and intolerable agony, the throat spasm would relax and respiration again become free. These attacks have occurred at very irregular intervals, sometimes several months apart, but generally two or three on successive or neighboring nights.

Borderlands of Migraine

Gowers (1907), in his preface to a series of lectures on "The Borderland of Epilepsy," announced his intention to speak of attacks which were *near* epilepsy, but not of it. He was concerned with the consideration of faints, vagal attacks, vertigo, sleep symptoms, and, above all, migraine. Epilepsies, in their most clearly recognizable form, are characterized by suddenness, brevity, loss of consciousness. But let us imagine, argues Gower,

. . . a minor epileptic attack that is extended, its elements protracted with no tendency to be terminated by loss of consciousness; its features would be so different that its nature would not be suspected.

It is indeed in these terms, as extended epilepsies, that Gowers would categorize many of the attacks he describes. He quotes, for example, the following case history as exemplifying a *vagal attack* akin to epilepsy:

The subject . . . was a man, an officer in the army, aged 30. The seizures were not frequent; they had occurred about once in six months for twelve years, ever since he was 18 years old. Earlier in the day he had been in especially good spirits—an antecedent often noted. Quite suddenly a dreamy mental state came on, a reminiscent state, the well-known feeling that whatever was happening had happened before. It was not momentary, as in epilepsy, but continued. With it, or just after its commencement, his hands and feet became cold. . . . With the coldness his face became increasingly pale, and physical prostration set in, speedily reaching such a degree that he was scarcely able to move. If he tried to sit up, he fell back at once. His extremities became icily cold, even to an observer. So great was the prostration that he could only utter one or two words at a time. . . . His pulse became smaller and smaller, until it was hardly perceptible. There was not a moment's loss of consciousness throughout. His own sensation was that he was dying, passing out of physical existence. The state lasted about half an hour, and then he became aware, simultaneously, that his mental state was improving and that his feet were a little less cold. The amelioration went on, but two or three minutes after its commencement a distinct rigor set in, with shivering and chattering of the teeth. . . . A few minutes after the rigor an urgent need for micturition was felt and went on during the rest of the day, a large quantity of limpid urine being passed. . . . He continued pale for the rest of the day.

The reader will recognize a large number of symptoms we have hitherto termed *migrainous* in this admirably detailed description. The antecedent feeling of well-being, the duration of the attack, its termination with a protracted diuresis, are all features we have encountered in the sequence of common migraines. By what warrant, therefore, is such an attack to be termed an extended epilepsy rather than a quite brief and severe, let us say, *condensed* migraine?

Virtually all the patterns of migraine equivalent we have considered in this chapter may present themselves in a more contracted format. Lennox and Lennox (1960) provide many instructive case histories under the title of autonomic or diencephalic epilepsy. Sometimes such autonomic attacks may evolve from or into clear-cut epilepsies or migraines, and at other times they may alternate with such attacks.

An obvious and important type of attack which bears obvious clinical affinities to both migraines and epilepsies—in terms of its widespread autonomic features to the former, and in terms of its suddenness and loss of consciousness to the latter—is the *faint*. Fainting not uncommonly coexists with recurrent migraine, and may occur with much the same periodicity as, or in similar provocative circumstances to, the migraine attacks. One may observe, as with vagal attacks, a continuous transition in the clinical picture from a dramatic and sudden collapse to protracted autonomic reactions with haziness, but not loss, of consciousness. The still briefer attacks which Gowers considers—vertigos, narcolepsies, cataplexies, and so on—will be considered in the next chapter, for their affinities are to migraine aura rather than common migraine and the migraine equivalents we have so far discussed.

Acute attacks of this type which are near migraine, but not of it, we may term *migranoid attacks*, and like migraine they tend to be periodic, recurrent, and strongly familial. We may reserve the term *migranoid reactions* for certain types of response akin to migraine in their clinical aspects, but circumstantially provoked rather than spontaneous and periodic. Here we must place the hyperbolic reactions to *heat* (and fever), *exhaustion, passive motion,* and certain *drugs* which are both common and characteristic in migraine patients. The distinction of what is a migraine and what a migranoid reaction is purely one of convenience. Thus it is awkward to call *motion-sickness* a migraine attack, but we may very conveniently term it a migranoid reaction, and note, in support of its affinities, that a large minority (almost fifty percent, according to Selby and Lance) of adult migraine sufferers experienced severe motion-sickness in childhood. Similarly a *hangover*—with its vascular headache, malaise, lethargy, nausea, and penitential depression—is usefully considered as a migranoid reaction; many migraine patients are highly intolerant of alcohol, and may suffer a spectrum of symptoms in its wake, from an acute nausea or headache reaction, to a full-blown hangover the following day. Feverish headaches and autonomic reactions may similarly be accounted migranoid in quality.

Similarly, there is a spectrum of drug responses, acute and sub-acute, characterized by diffuse central and autonomic reactions, akin both to syncopal and to migraine attacks. Thus, the following description of a "nitritoid crisis" is cited by Goodman and Gilman (1955):

Normal robust male, aged 28, given 0.18 gm of sodium nitrite by mouth. . . . Yawning appeared and became progressively more prominent; the respirations deepened and assumed a sighing character; restlessness, belching and borborygmus were noted; and a cold perspiration broke out over the entire body surface. In about twenty minutes the skin was ashen grey, the subject became drowsy . . . the blood pressure reading became unobtainable . . . and unconsciousness ensued.

Reactions of a similar acuteness may occur following visceral dilatation or injury, reflex or hemorrhagic fall of blood pressure, toxic and metabolic insults (e.g. hypoglycemia), and in allergic and anaphylactoid responses.

We will have to concern ourselves later with the question of whether such responses afford useful "models" of the migraine reaction, and content ourselves, at this point, with noting their clinical affinity and place in the borderlands of migraine.

Alternations and Concomitances with other Disorders

Even more complicated than these cases in which two allied symptoms alternate, are those patients who present with a *polymorphous* syndrome in which a large variety of symptoms—with clinical and physiological affinities to each other—occur simultaneously or cyclically in the history of the individual:

Case 49

This 31-year-old engineer has already been cited in connection with a tendency to postprandial stupors. He suffers from a variety of further symptoms, as follows:

(a) A continuous "latent" vascular headache, which becomes manifest on stooping, jolting, or coughing.
(b) Attacks of common migraine.
(c) Night sweats, for which no organic basis has been found.
(d) Attacks of nocturnal salivation.
(e) Attacks of abdominal pain and diarrhea—contrast studies of the bowel have always been negative.
(f) Orthostatic hypotension.
(g) Occasional sleep-paralysis, narcolepsy, and cataplexy.

He is otherwise in excellent health.

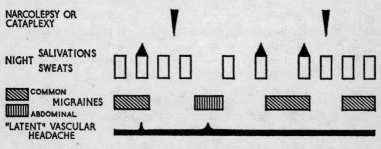

Figure 1a. Case 49

Case 75

A 35-year-old physician subject to migraine auras and classical migraine has also experienced, as alternative reactions, abdominal migraines, bilious attacks, stuporous migraine equivalents, "vagal attacks" (exceedingly similar in type to that described by Gowers), and, more rarely, fainting and narcolepsy. All of these reactions are circumstantially determined, either by exhaustion or acute emotional stress, especially if these factors are conjoined. He cannot predict *which* somatic response will occur: all of them seem equally available and equivalent to one another.

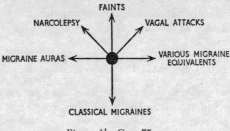

Figure 1b. Case 75

Case 64

A polysymptomatic woman of 45 with the following history: Intrinsic (usually nocturnal) asthma until the age of 20, recurrent duodenal ulceration between the ages of 20 and 37. At the age of 38 she had an initial episode of rheumatoid arthritis, and has had several episodes subsequently. Coincident with the inauguration of this symptom, she started to have frequent attacks of angioneurotic edema and of common migraine. These two latter syndromes have coalesced, and since the age of 43 her attacks of migraine have been ushered in by facial and periocular edema.

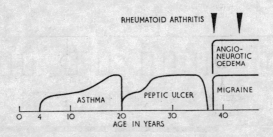

Figure 1c. Case 64

Case 62

A 51-year-old woman whose social and emotional history will be elaborated in Part II. She had suffered for more than twenty years with three somatic manifestations: common migraine, ulcerative colitis, and psoriasis. She would suffer for several months from one of these symptoms, before remitting and passing to another symptom. She was thus trapped within an endless malignant cycle.

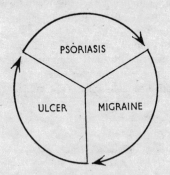

Figure 1d. Case 62

Case 61

A 38-year-old woman who presented herself for treatment of common migraine, although she also had disfiguring psoriasis. Her family background was one of polymorphous functional disease: migraine, hayfever, asthma, urticaria, Menière's disease, peptic ulcer, ulcerative colitis, and Crohn's disease. It was difficult to avoid the feeling that this stricken family was, in effect, committing physiological suicide.

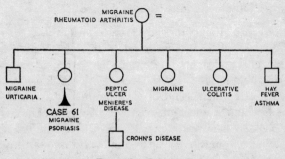

Figure 1e. Case 61

Case 21

A highly intelligent 25-year-old woman who combines several neurotic symptoms with a variety of somatic syndromes. She had had classical migraines since childhood, of which there is a prominent family history: the majority of these attacks arise at dawn with a nightmare or night-terror—the figments of nightmare and unmistakable scotomatous figures may be coalesced, prior to her waking in the second, or headache, stage. On some occasions, the aura is followed by abdominal pain but no head pain. Allied to the latter, but missing an aura, are pre-menstrual syndromes, in which a period of water-retention, constipation, and restlessness deliquesces into diuresis, diarrhea, and menstrual flux: there may or may not be an associated vascular headache with these premenstrual syndromes. On some occasions she has had "grey outs," or syncopes, usually though not invariably followed by migrainous headache. She is also subject to attacks of urticaria (hives) during periods of increased emotional stress. With successful treatment of her headache problems, the emphasis has shifted to increased abdominal attacks and urticaria.

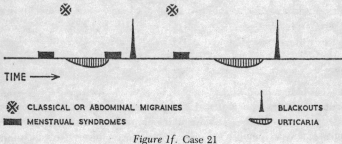

TIME ——→

�֎ CLASSICAL OR ABDOMINAL MIGRAINES   ⏐ BLACKOUTS

▨ MENSTRUAL SYNDROMES   ⏝ URTICARIA

Figure 1f. Case 21

Differential Diagnosis and Nomenclature

When the cardinal symptom of vascular headache is absent, the types of attack we have considered in this chapter may present formidable challenges in differential diagnosis; indeed, there is probably no field in medicine so strewn with the debris of misdiagnosis and mistreatment, and of well-intentioned but wholly mistaken medical and surgical interventions. Abdominal migraines, for example, no less than wasting crises, must have afforded innumerable occasions for emergency laparotomies. It may not be justifiable to wait passively for the outcome of a mysterious but overwhelming attack of abdominal pain; it is doubtless better sense to perform a negative laparotomy in a case of abdominal migraine than be faced with a neglected appendicitis and peritonitis. The true diagnosis may only become apparent subsequently, with repetition of the attacks, and demonstration of their benign and transient nature. In many cases, therefore, the diagnosis of cryptic migraine equivalents requires prolonged observation, and may, in fact, be made only retrospectively.

We have limited our consideration, thus far, to relatively distinct, circumscribed, and strongly marked paroxysmal attacks, and have selected, for the sake of emphasis, case histories of an almost diagrammatic clarity. In practice, the symptoms experienced and the history obtainable may be altogether vaguer in terms of specific symptoms. Attacks characterized by little more than malaise are likely to be regarded as mild viral illnesses. Attacks characterized by alteration of affect and consciousness—mild drowsiness or depression—may be taken for purely emotional reactions. Both viral illnesses and emotional reaction *may*, indeed, share many clinical symptoms occurring in, though not pathognomonic of, migraines, and the differential diagnosis may never be clarified unless more specific symptoms, or determinants of the attacks, are elicited.

Beyond the sharp and artificial edges of "diagnosis" we enter a region of semantic ambiguity in which the definition of the term *migraine* is stretched to the breaking point. In the center, so to speak, we may place common migraine, clear and indisputable. Around this we may group the migraine equivalents, polymorphous in their manifestations, and representing various dissections, decompositions, and agglomerates of different migraine components. Beyond this, we must recognize a penumbra of allied and analogous reactions, which may, as it were, do duty for a migraine.

Compact and clearly defined at its center, migraine diffuses outward until it merges with an immense surrounding field of allied phenomena. The only boundaries which exist are those which we are forced to adopt for nosological clarity and clinical action. We construct such boundaries and limits, for there are none in the subject itself.

It should be emphasized that though for purposes of exposition and analysis, we may present migraine as a list or aggregate of symptoms, or speak of migraine as a sort of syndrome or composite, this is not how it presents itself to the suffering patient. For him it is entry into a strange and sick world, an unmistakable but unanalyzable feeling that "something is wrong." This is expressed by du Bois Reymond, when he speaks of each attack starting with "a general feeling of disorder." Experience teaches the migraine patient that this general, discordant, morbid feeling is, in fact, the first intimation of a migraine—the first apprehension of its peculiar *landscape*. As he enters deeper into this dread landscape, it reveals more and more features, the whole physiognomy, the *face*, of migraine.

3

Migraine Aura and
Classical Migraine

Introduction

We now come to the largest, strangest chapter in this book—for we
must consider what lies at the very heart of migraine; here is the
realm of its great wonders and secrets:

We carry with us the wonders we seek without us: there is all Africa and
her prodigies in us. . . .

Sir Thomas Browne's words perfectly fit this—the *aura* of migraine:
here, inside us, is a veritable Africa of prodigies; here, by experience, exploration and reflection, one can chart a whole world—the
cosmography of oneself.

The aura of migraine deserves a whole book to itself—or, at the
very least, as in Liveing, it should form the centerpiece if a book is
to be written on migraine. But, very puzzlingly, the reverse obtains;
nobody has given the aura its due, since Liveing; and the more up-
to-date the book, the less space it is given. The very words we
use—*classical* migraine as opposed to *common* (the *classical* being
a migraine with an aura)—imply that the aura is *uncommon*—and
arcane.

This, as a start, is demonstrably untrue, and a consequence of
inquiries which fly wide of the mark, and foolish assumptions which
make them miss the mark. An acute and open-minded observer
like Alvarez, putting together the experience of seventy years
as a physician, considered the aura was far commoner than usually

allowed; far commoner, indeed, than anything else in a migraine. And in this I find myself in complete agreement with him.

The following general points should first be made by way of introduction.

The aura itself is far from uncommon; adequate descriptions of it are extremely uncommon; good descriptions of the aura are vitally *needed*, because it is a phenomenon of the utmost importance, which can cast a great flood of light not only on migraine, but on the most elemental and fundamental mechanisms of the brain-mind; good descriptions are hard to obtain, because many aura phenomena are exceedingly strange—so strange as to transcend the powers of language; and good descriptions are made rarer still by the presence of something uncanny and fearful, the very thought of which causes the mind to shy.

This last, although neither analyzed nor understood, was given a very striking emphasis by Liveing; it constituted a strange and incomprehensible barrier, over which neither he nor his patients could leap; so that, finally he could only say that "there are sufferers who cannot bear to think or talk of their attacks, and always refer to them with horror, though this is clearly not on account of the pain they occasion." Thus the subject of migraine aura is touched with the incomprehensible and the incommunicable: nay, this lies at its very center, its heart.

The term *aura* has been used for nearly two thousand years to denote the sensory hallucinations immediately preceding certain epileptic seizures.* The term has been employed, for somewhat over a century, to denote analogous symptoms which inaugurate certain attacks—the so-called classical migraine—or which may constitute, on occasion, the sole manifestation of a migraine attack.

We will have occasion to consider, as components of these auras, symptoms of an acuteness and a strangeness which sets them apart

---

*The derivation and original meaning of the term is described by Gowers as follows: "The word *aura* was first used by Pelops, the master of Galen, who was struck by the phenomenon with which many attacks begin—a sensation, commencing in the hand or foot, apparently ascending to the head. The sensation having been described to him by patients as 'a cold vapor,' he suggested that it might really be such, passing up the vessels, then believed to contain air. Hence he named it πνευματικὴ αὔρα 'spirituous vapor.'"

from anything we have thus far discussed. Indeed, if an aura were never followed by vascular headache, nausea, diffuse autonomic disturbance, and other phenomena, we might have great difficulty in recognizing its migrainous nature. Such difficulties *do* arise, not uncommonly, when patients suffer from isolated auras lasting a few minutes, and not succeeded by headache or vegetative disturbance. Such cases, as Gowers remarked, are very puzzling, of great importance, and liable to be misunderstood.

Such uncertainties are reflected in a historical dichotomy, whereby accounts of (migraine) aura and accounts of (migraine) headache were separately published for centuries, without the making of any explicit connection between the two sets of phenomena.

The manifestations of migraine aura are exceedingly various, and include not only simple and complex sensory hallucinations but intense affective states, deficits and disturbances of speech and ideation, dislocations of space- and time-perception, and a variety of dreamy, delirious, and trancelike states. The older medical and religious literature contains innumerable references to "visions," "trances," "transports," and other occurrences, but the nature of many of these must now remain enigmatic to us. Many different processes may have similar manifestations, and some of the more complex phenomena described may be hysteric, psychotic, oneiric, or hypnagogic in origin, no less than epileptic, apoplectic, toxic, or migrainous in nature.

A single notable exception may be mentioned—the "visions" of Hildegard (1098–1179)—which were indisputably migrainous in nature. These are discussed in an appendix to this chapter.

Isolated accounts of such visual phenomena continued to appear throughout the Middle Ages, but we must move six hundred years before we find accounts of aura phenomena other than the visual, and the making of an *explicit* connection between such manifestations and migraine.

The following three accounts, all written in the early nineteenth century, and cited by Liveing, illustrate many cardinal characteristics of migraine aura, in its visual (scotomatous), tactile (paresthetic), and aphasic forms. We may note, parenthetically, that many of the finest descriptions of the aura—from those of Hildegard in the twelfth century to those of Lashley and Alvarez in the present century—have been provided by introspective observers who themselves suffered from classical migraine, or, more commonly, isolated migraine auras.

I have frequently experienced a sudden failure of sight. The general sight did not appear affected; but when I looked at any particular object, it seemed as if something brown, and more or less opaque, was interposed between my eyes and it, so that I saw it indistinctly, or sometimes not at all. . . .

After it had continued a few moments, the upper or lower edge appeared bounded by an edging of light of a zigzag shape, and coruscating nearly at right angles to its length. The coruscation always appeared to be in one eye; but both it and the cloud existed equally whether I looked at an object with one or both eyes open. . . . The cloud and the coruscation . . . would remain from twenty minutes, sometimes to half an hour. . . . They were in me never followed by headache . . . [but] generally went off with a movement in the stomach producing eructation.

—Parry

Commencing in the tip of the tongue, at one part of the face, at the ends of the fingers or toes, it [the paraesthesia] mounts little by little towards the cerebrospinal axis, successively disappearing about those parts where it was first developed. . . . The thrilling sensation in the hands calls to mind the oscillatory movement of the visual image.

—Piorry

About a quarter of an hour after this [the blindness], she feels a numbness of the little finger of the right hand, beginning at the point of it, and extending very gradually over the whole hand and arm, producing a complete loss of sensibility of the parts, but without any loss of the power of motion. The feeling of numbness then extends to the right side of the head, and from this it seems to spread downwards towards the stomach. When it reaches the side of the head, she becomes oppressed and partially confused, answers questions slowly and confusedly, and her speech is considerably affected; when it reaches the stomach she sometimes vomits.

—Abercrombie

The elective sites of the paresthesiae (tongue, hand, foot), and its centripetal passage from the periphery, necessarily reminded the early observers of the *aura epileptica,* and it remained for Liveing, writing between 1863 and 1865, to make an absolutely clear distinction between the two sets of phenomena.

Our next task must be a systematic enumeration of the full range of aural symptoms which may occur. Since they are exceedingly various, we may consider them under certain general heads:

(a) Specific visual, tactile, and other sensory hallucinations.
(b) General alterations of sensory threshold and excitability.
(c) Alterations in level of consciousness and muscular tone.
(d) Alterations of mood and affect.
(e) Disorders of higher integrative functions: perception, ideation, memory, and speech.

These categories are adopted purely for ease of discussion. They are in no sense mutually exclusive. Migraine aura, like common migraine, is composite in nature, and put together from a variety of possible components. Although a casual description may make reference to a single symptom only, such as a scintillating scotoma, a patient interrogation will nearly always reveal that the situation is more complex, and that several phenomena—some very subtle, and difficult of description—are happening simultaneously.

We shall first enumerate individual components of the aura point by point, remembering that they are isolated only for purposes of exposition. This will be followed by a series of case histories designed to illustrate the complex and composite nature of auras as they usually occur.

Specific Sensory Hallucinations: Visual

A remarkable variety of visual hallucinations may be experienced during the course of a migraine aura.

The simplest hallucination takes the form of a dance of brilliant stars, sparks, flashes, or simple geometric forms across the visual field. Phosphenes of this type are usually white, but may have brilliant spectral colors. They may number many hundreds, and swarm rapidly across the visual field (patients often compare them to the movement of radar "blips" across a screen). Sometimes a single phosphene may detach itself from the remainder, as in the following case (Gowers, 1892):

One patient . . . with characteristic headaches preceded by hemianopia, complained of bright stars before the eyes whenever she had looked at a brilliant light; and sometimes one of the stars, brighter than the rest, would start from the right lower corner of the field of vision, and pass across the field, generally quickly, in a second, sometimes more slowly, and when it reached the left side would break up and leave a blue area in which luminous points were moving.*

At other times there may only be a single, rather elaborate phosphene in the visual field, which moves to and fro upon a set course, and then disappears suddenly, leaving a trail of dazzlement or blindness in its wake (*figure 2a*). We may, once more, find the best descriptions of such phosphenes among Gowers' many writings on the subject (1904).

In another case a radial movement was presented by a stellate object which remained unchanged throughout. It appeared usually near the edge of the right half of the field just below the horizontal line, and consisted of about six pointed leaflike projections, alternately red and blue . . . [it] moved slowly towards the left and upwards, passing above the fixing-point, to a little beyond the middle line, then it returned to its starting place, retraced this path once or twice, and then passed to the right edge of the field . . . after two or three repetitions of the last course it suddenly disappeared . . . [on opening her eyes] the patient always found she could only see in the part of the field through which the spectrum had not passed.

Although such phosphenes may be confined to one half or one quadrant of the visual field, they not infrequently cross the midline (as in the case described above); rapidly moving swarms of phosphenes are bilateral more often than not. Sometimes the phosphenes may be elaborated or interpreted by the patient as recognizable images; thus one patient (in Selby and Lance's series) described small white skunks with erect tails, moving in procession across one quadrant of the visual field.**

*This case history also draws attention to the specific capacity of light to provoke various forms of migraine aura, a subject more fully discussed in chapter 8.

**Hughlings Jackson makes the following comment on the tendency to elaborate images from elementary hallucinations when in physiologically abnormal states: "A healthy man has muscae from intra-ocular specks; they seem like moving dots and films in front of him. But suppose he undergoes dissolution (as in cases of delirium tremens), and that there is the first depth of dissolution, then he sees mice and rats. Speaking roughly, the muscae 'turn into' those animals for him."

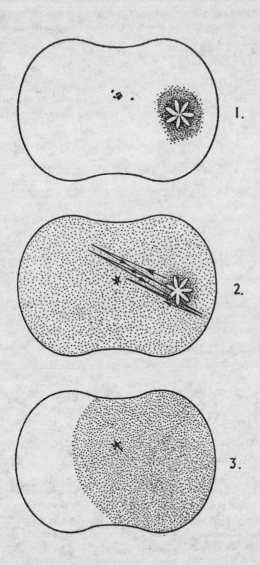

Figure 2a. Variants of migraine scotoma; reproduced from Gowers
(1904); mobile stellate spectrum

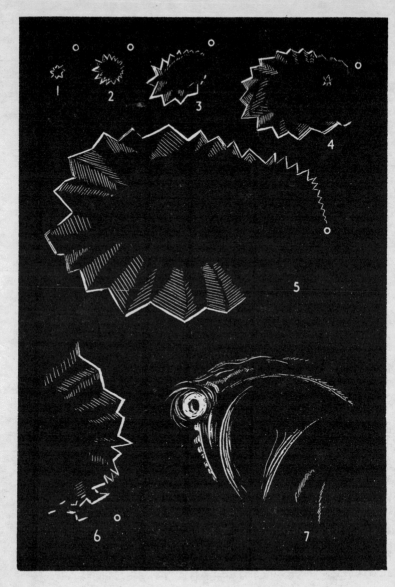

Figure 2b. Variants of migraine scotoma; reproduced from Gowers (1904); expanding angular spectrum (Airy, 1868)

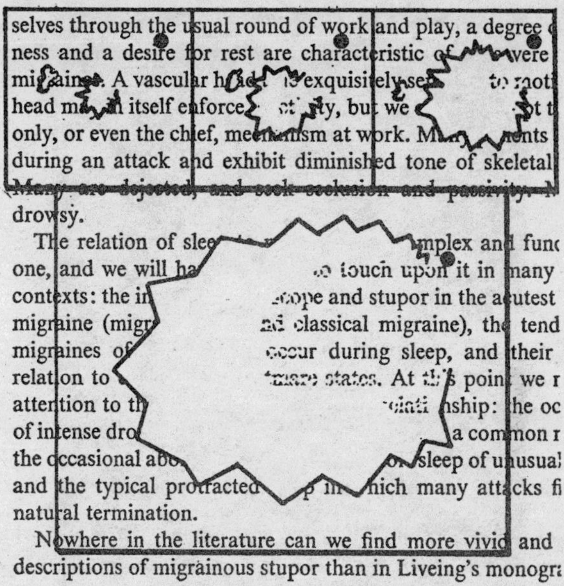

selves through the usual round of work and play, a degree
ness and a desire for rest are characteristic of ... were
migraine. A vascular h... exquisitely se... to moti
head m... in itself enforce... ...ly, but we ...t t
only, or even the chief, mechanism at work. M... ...ents
during an attack and exhibit diminished tone of skeletal
... ...
drowsy.

The relation of slee... ...mplex and func
one, and we will ha... ...o touch upon it in many
contexts: the i... ...cope and stupor in the acutest
migraine (migr... ...d classical migraine), the tend
migraines of ... ...occur during sleep, and their
relation to ... ...ture states. At th's point we r
attention to t... ...ti nship: he oc
of intense dro... ...a common r
the occasional ab... ...sleep of unusual
and the typical protracted ... p in which many attacks fi
natural termination.

Nowhere in the literature can we find more vivid and
descriptions of migrainous stupor than in Liveing's monogra

Figure 2c. Variants of migraine scotoma; after Gowers
(1904); expanding negative scotoma

Other elementary hallucinations which are commonly experienced are rippling, shimmering and undulation in the visual field,
which patients may compare to the appearance of wind-blown water,
or looking though watered silk. (See *figure 6a* and *6b*.)

During or after the passage of simple phosphenes, some patients
may observe, on closing the eyes, a form of visual tumult or
delirium, in which latticed, faceted and tessellated motifs predomi-
nate—images reminiscent of mosaics, honeycombs, Turkish carpets,
and so on, or moiré patterns. These figments and elementary images
tend to be brilliantly luminous, colored, highly unstable, and prone
to sudden kaleidoscopic transformations.

These evanescent flitting phosphenes are usually no more than a
preamble to the major portion of the visual aura. In most (though
not all) cases the patient goes on to experience a longer-lasting
and far more elaborate hallucination within the visual field—the
migraine *scotoma*. Further descriptive terms are commonly used:
the shape (and colors) of these scotomata lead us to speak of migraine

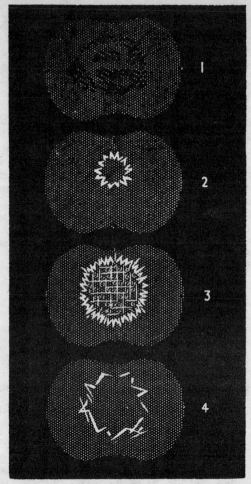

Figure 2d. Variants of migraine scotoma; reproduced from Gowers
(1904); pericentral spectrum

spectra, and the structure of their margins (often reminiscent of the
ramparts of a walled city) has given rise to the term *fortification
spectra* (teichopsia). The term *scintillating scotoma* denotes the
characteristic flickering of luminous migraine spectra, and the term
negative scotoma denotes the area of partial or total blindness which
may follow, or, on occasion, precede a scintillating scotoma.

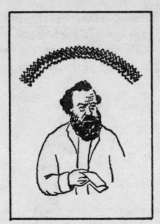

Figure 2e. Variants of migraine scotoma; reproduced from Gowers
(1904); rainbow spectrum

The majority of migraine scotomata present as a sudden brilliant
luminosity near the fixation-point in one visual half-field; from here
the scotoma generally expands and moves slowly toward the edge
of the visual field, assuming the form of a giant crescent or horse-
shoe. Its subjective brightness is blinding—Lashley compares it to
that of a white surface in noonday sunlight. Within this brilliance
there may be a play of intense, pure spectral colors at the fringes
of the scotoma, and objects seen through these fringes may be
edged with a many-colored iridescence. The advancing margin of
the scotoma often displays the gross zigzag appearance which
justifies the term *fortification-spectrum* (*figure 2b*), and is invariably
broken up, more finely, into minute luminous angles and intersecting lines—this *cheveux de frise* is particularly well shown in
Lashley's sketches and is coarser in the lower portions of the scotoma
(*figure 3*). There is a characteristic boiling movement or scintillation
throughout the luminous portions of the scotoma: the effect is vividly
conveyed in a nineteenth-century description:

It may be likened to the effect produced by the rapid gyration of small
waterbeetles as they are seen swarming in a cluster on the surface of the
water in sunshine . . .

The rate of scintillation is below the flicker-fusion-frequency, yet
too fast to count; its frequency has been estimated, by indirect

methods, as lying between eight and twelve scintillations per second. The margin of the scintillating scotoma advances at a rather constant rate, and usually takes between ten and twenty minutes to pass from the neighborhood of the fixation-point to the edge of the visual field (*figure 3b*).

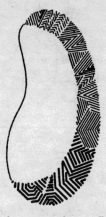

Figure 3a. Course and structure of a scintillating scotoma; from Lashley (1941); fine structure of intersecting lines (*cheveux de frise*) at advancing border of scintillating scotoma

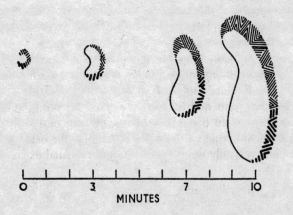

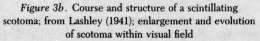

Figure 3b. Course and structure of a scintillating scotoma; from Lashley (1941); enlargement and evolution of scotoma within visual field

Perhaps the most detailed figures and descriptions ever given of migraine scotomata are those of Airy (1868); these are reproduced in detail both by Liveing and Gowers, and may without apology be cited once again. The stages of Airy's scotomata are shown in *figure 2b*.

A bright stellate object, a small angled sphere, suddenly appears in one side of the combined field . . . it rapidly enlarges, first as a circular zigzag, but on the inner side, toward the medial line, the regular outline becomes faint, and, as the increase in size goes on, the outline here becomes broken, the gap becoming larger as the whole increases, and the original circular outline becomes oval. The form assumed is roughly concentric with the edge of the field of vision . . . the lines which constitute the outline meet at right angles or larger angles. . . . When this angled oval has extended through the greater part of the half-field the upper portion expands; it seems to overcome at last some resistance in the immediate neighborhood of the fixing point . . . so that a bulge occurs in the part above, and the angular elements of the outline here enlarge. . . . After this final stage occurs, the outer part of the outline disappears. This final expansion near the center progresses with great rapidity, and ends in a whirling center of light from which sprays of light seem flying off. Then all is over, and the headache comes on.

Elsewhere Airy speaks of the rapid "boiling and trembling motion," and the "bastioned" outline of the scotoma (he suggested the name "teichopsia"); he speaks of the "gorgeous chromatic edgings" to the figure, a spectacle marred for him only by the anticipation of ensuing headache.

The margins of the luminous scotoma trail behind them a shadow-crescent of total blindness, behind which is a penumbral region where visual excitability is in process of restoration (*figures 2c and 3a*). Airy also makes reference (and the symptom is not an uncommon one) to the occasional appearance of a second scintillating focus following within a few minutes of the original scotoma, that is, immediately upon the restitution of visual excitability near the fixation point.

Such is the sequence in the commonest type of migraine scotoma (the expanding angular spectrum of Gowers); there may occur, however, many important variations on this theme, the existence of which must be taken into account if any adequate theory of the scotoma is to be derived. Not all scotomata commence near the fixation point; a number of patients consistently, and a few occasionally, experience scotomata starting eccentrically or peripherally in the visual field (Gowers' radial spectra). Expanding scotomata may appear alternately or simultaneously in both half-fields, and their continued alternation, in the former case, may give rise to an aura "status" lasting hours. Of great theoretical importance (and especial aesthetic appeal) are those bilateral scotomata whose evolution is exactly synchronized in both half-fields—the central and pericentral spectra of Gowers (*figure 2d*). The existence of such scotomata poses very difficult problems to those who postulate a local, one-sided process as the basis of migraine auras.*

Luminous or negative scotomata may be not only central, but quadrantic, altitudinal or irregular in their distribution. A particularly pleasing pattern is that of a spectrum in the form of an arch, centrally and bilaterally placed in the visual field (*figure 2e*); Gowers considers these to be segments of a pericentral spectrum. Such a spectrum was described by Aretaeus nearly two thousand years ago, and compared by him to the appearance of a rainbow in the sky.

A *negative* scotoma generally follows a scintillating scotoma, but occasionally precedes it, and sometimes occurs in its stead. In the latter event, as with all manifestations of cortical blindness, it may be discovered by accident, for example, by suddenly observing the bisection of a face, or the disappearance of certain words or figures on a page. It is important to note, however, that observant patients consistently allude to a special "dazzled" quality which appears to be an innate characteristic of negative scotomata. In the words of an old description cited by Liveing:

My sight suddenly becomes disordered, more on one side than the other, like a person who has looked at the sun.

We cannot refrain from contrasting this "dazzled" quality with the "blinding" brilliance of the scintillation if it occurs. The suspicion arises that the extinction of vision and visual excitability may not, after all, be a primary phenomenon, but a consequence of some

---

*Gowers, speaking of central negative scotomata, states: "Such a central loss, so perfectly symmetrical, seems inexplicable by an assumed disturbance of the function of one hemisphere. It can only be explained . . . by a simultaneous functional inhibition (of both hemispheres), perfectly symmetrical."

preceding excitation affecting the nonvisual areas of the brain. This hypothesis will be explored later, and we may simply take note, at this stage, of descriptions which *do* indicate some such antecedent excitation:

Case 67

A 32-year-old physician who has had classical migraines and isolated auras since childhood. The scotomata are always negative, but appear to be preceded by a type of analeptic excitation. In the patient's words: "It starts with a sort of excited feeling, as if I had taken an amphetamine. I know that something is happening to me, and I start to look around. I wonder if there is something the matter with the light. Then I notice that part of my visual field is missing."

Here we see that a negative scotomata can occur during and despite persistent analeptic excitement; other patients show the converse— scintillating scotomata associated with intense drowsiness. In such cases there is a *paradoxical concurrence of excitation and inhibition*.

It should be evident from the many references to it in this book and the many illustrations that the phenomena of *scotoma* were considered of the most central importance. And yet—it is now clear to me—I dealt with these inadequately in 1970; I made omissions— indeed, a central omission; I may say that I omitted the very center of the subject—or (to make a play on words) that I exhibited a *scotoma* in my understanding of *scotoma*.

The Angst of Scotoma

A peculiar *horror*—perhaps this is part of the horror of which Liveing speaks—may be associated with negative scotomata, which may be felt, not just as a failure of sight but a failure of reality itself.

This feeling, full of fear and deeply uncanny, is indicated in the following case histories:

Case 77

A highly gifted physician, a psychoanalyst, who has had occasional negative scotomata, or hemianopia, coming two or three times a year since early childhood. These are frequently, but not invariably, followed by migraine headaches.

Although this man is taken daily into the depths of the soul and its primeval terrors by his calling and profession, and although he boldly faces all the monsters of the unconscious, he has never become inured to his own scotomata, which introduce a realm or category of the unbearable and uncanny, beyond anything he has encountered in the realms of psychiatry. In his own words:

"I may be seeing as a patient someone I know well, sitting across the desk, with my gaze fixed upon them. Suddenly I become aware that something is wrong—although at this point I cannot say what it is. It is a sense of something *fundamentally* wrong—something impossible and contrary to the order of nature.

Then I suddenly 'realize'—*part of the patient's face is missing:* part of their nose, or their cheek, or perhaps the left ear. Although I continue to listen and speak, my gaze seems transfixed—I cannot move my head—and a sense of horror, of the impossible, steals over me. The disappearance continues—usually until half the face has disappeared and, with this, that same half of the room. I feel paralyzed and petrified in some sort of way. It never occurs to me that something is happening to my vision—I feel something incredible is happening to the *world*. It doesn't occur to me to move my head or eyes to 'check' on the existence of what seems to be missing. It never occurs to me that I am having a migraine, even though I have had the experience dozens of times before. . . .

I don't exactly feel that anything is 'missing,' but I fall into a ridiculous obsessive doubt. I seem to lose the *idea* of a face; I 'forget' how faces look—something happens to my imagination, my memory, my thinking. . . . It is not that half the world mysteriously 'disappears,' but that I find myself in doubt as to whether it was ever there. There seems to be a sort of hole in my memory and mind and, so to speak, a hole in the world; and yet I cannot imagine what might go in the hole. There is a hole and there isn't a hole—my mind is utterly confounded. I have the feeling that my body—that *bodies* are unstable, that they may come apart and lose parts of themselves—an eye, a limb, amputation—that something vital has disappeared, but disappeared *without trace*, that it has disappeared *along with the 'place' it once occupied*. The horrible feeling is of nothingness nowhere.*

After a while—perhaps it is only a minute or two, but it seems to last

---

*Compare Hobbes: "That which is not Body is no part of the Universe . . . and since the Universe is All . . . that which is not Body is Nothing . . . and Nowhere." Hobbes, *The Kingdome of Darknesse*.

forever—I realize that there is something wrong with my vision, that it is a natural, physiological disturbance in my vision, and not some grotesque, unnatural disturbance in the world. I realize that I am having a migraine aura—and an immense sense of relief floods over me. . . .

But even knowing this does not *correct* the perception. . . . There is still a certain residue of dread, and a fear that the scotoma may go on forever. . . . It is only when there is full restoration of the visual fields that the sense of panic, and of something wrong, finally goes away. . . .

I have never experienced this sort of fear except in regard to a migraine scotoma."

Case 78

This woman of 75 has frequent attacks—variously called "migraine auras" or "epilepsies" or sometimes "migralepsies"—which have a clear physiological basis in a discharging lesion, a scar, in her right parietoccipital area due to an injury sustained in infancy.

In these attacks the left side of her body seems to disappear and everything normally seen on the left disappears. She says: "There is nothing there any more, just a blank, just a hole"—a blank in her visual field, in her body, in the universe itself, and in that state she cannot trust herself to stand, and must sit down before it gets worse. She also experiences a feeling of mortal terror when she has these attacks. She feels the "hole" is like death, and that one day it will get so large that it will "swallow" her completely. She had these attacks as a child but was called a "liar" when she described them.

In severe attacks, it is not only the left side of her body which seems to disappear, but she is deeply confused about her *whole* body, and cannot be sure where anything is—or *that* it is.

She feels quite unreal (this is one of the reasons for her fears of engulfment). Also in such severe attacks she cannot make sense of what she *can* see (visual agnosia) and, specifically, she may be unable to recognize the faces of familiar people—either their faces seem "different" or, more commonly, they seem "faceless," for example, they have features which bear no expression (prosopagnosia). In the worst attacks this extends to voices too—they are heard, but lose all tonality and "character"; a sort of auditory agnosia.

Such privations of sense go on to complete darkness and silence—as in cases recorded by Gowers—and she might be said to lose consciousness, although essentially it is a dissolution of her sensorium in which she gradually sinks to deeper and deeper "senselessness" until finally she is completely insensible. It is not surprising that attacks so dreadful and so real are experienced as deathlike.

The word *scotoma* means darkness or shadow, and we can understand from the above history something of the quality of this shadow. In the case of *bilateral* scotoma, there may be even more horrifying experiences; thus a bilateral, central scotoma causes the middle of the visual field, the world, to disappear—and faces, at such times, have the center punched out, and become a ring of flesh surrounding a void (a condition termed *doughnut* or *bagel* vision).

If there is a complete bilateral scotoma, with total loss of the visual fields, and (as may happen, from the proximity of the visual and tactile areas in the brain) total loss of the body-fields, or sense of the body, a most terrifying sense of extermination may occur.

If one category of horror is annihilation—of vision, visibility, visuality, imagery, of a perceptible-or-imaginable world—the other, and more picturesque, is "visions" of all sorts, produced by excitations in the visual and imaginative apparatus. The simplest such "visions" are scintillations and phosphenes, but there are an infinity of more complex ones, some too strange, or too frightening, to communicate—so that patients maintain a secrecy or reserve, and may avoid speaking, or even thinking, about them. This is especially likely if the sufferers are children—and migraine aura is commonest of all in childhood. Cardan, in his autobiography, relates that in childhood he would sometimes see elves, which would dance in one half of the visual field, and disappear after 15 to 20 minutes; he adds that *he dared not mention this to anyone at all, lest he be thought insane, or a liar;* and that he himself was confounded by this "deception of the senses." Dr. J. C. Steele, working with migrainous children in Toronto, was able to persuade them to paint their aura-visions, or to collaborate with a medical artist; and on the basis of this work (which required remarkable sensitivity, patience, and empathy, working with very young, and often very scared children) he compiled an *atlas* of migrainous "visions." This atlas gives a wonderful idea of the variety and complexity of such "visions," and of the great illumination which they can cast on fundamental perceptual mechanisms—all the ways in which we "see" and construct reality; and of the countless other, phantasmal worlds—like the elf-world described by Cardan—which may also be constructed under the impetus of a strangely altered visual-imaginative physiology.

Dr. Steele indicated to me the immense relief which was shown by these "visionary" children when they were able to admit their strange experiences, and to encounter a friendly sympathetic understanding—instead of the tellings-off, the scoldings, they had previously met; they could now speak out, be listened to, and be understood.

The sense of violation, of the uncanny, of horror, only occurs if the situation is acute, and there is some remainder of the person to see what has happened (or, rather, what is no longer happening). A scotoma may be missed, even when acute, and with an acute observer—as, at first, in case 77. And it is almost invariably "missed" (the person fails to miss what is "missing") when it is long-standing, persistent, or chronic: a situation one not uncommonly sees with some strokes. The following case history illustrates this:

Case 79

An intelligent woman in her sixties who had suffered a massive stroke, affecting the deeper and back portions of her right cerebral hemisphere. She has perfectly preserved intelligence—and humor.

She sometimes complains to the nurses that they have not put dessert or coffee on her tray. . . . When they said: "But, Mrs. X, it is right there, on the left," she seems not to understand what they say, and does not look to the left. If her head is gently turned, so that the dessert comes into sight, in the preserved right half of her visual field, she says: "Oh there it is—it wasn't there before." She has totally lost the *idea* of "left," both with regard to the world, and also her own body. Sometimes she complains that her portions are too small—but this is because she only eats from the right half of the plate—it does not occur to her that it has a left half as well. Sometimes, she will put on lipstick, and make up the right half of her face, leaving the left half completely neglected: it is almost impossible to treat these things, because her attention cannot be drawn to them ("hemi-inattention"), and she has no conception that they are "wrong." She knows it intellectually, and can understand, and laugh; but it is impossible for her to know it *directly*.

Specific Tactile Hallucinations

Many of the observations which have been made with regard to the visual manifestations may be applied to the tactile hallucinations of migraine aura. There may be positive (paresthetic) or negative (anesthetic) hallucinations. The paresthesiae have a characteristic thrilling or vibrato of the same frequency as the visual scintillations. Tactile hallucinations may coexist with scotomata, precede them, follow them, or occur in their absence, although they are appreciably less common than the visual manifestations. There is no constancy in this, even in repeated attacks in the same patient.

They most commonly announce their appearance in the most excitable and massively represented portions of the tactile field—about the tongue and mouth, in the hand or hands, and less commonly in the feet—as the scotomata usually appear in relation to the macula or maculae of the visual field. Very occasionally they may start on the trunk, the thigh, or other portions of the tactile field.

Mild or fleeting paresthesiae may remain at their point of origin; more commonly they spread centripetally, from the distal to the proximal portions of the limbs. It is entirely legitimate, therefore, to compare them to the Jacksonian march of an epileptic aura, if we remember two important differences. The centripetal passage of migraine paresthesia, like that of scintillating scotomata, is far slower than the corresponding passage of epileptic paresthesia—a single "sweep" of the migraine aura occupies twenty to thirty minutes. Recurrent cycles of paresthesia may follow one another for hours on end, or alternate with cycles of scotomata, in a migraine "status." Secondly, in contradistinction to epileptic auras which start unilaterally in the vast majority of cases, the paresthesia of migraine aura start *bilaterally,* or become bilateral, in more than half of all the cases. Bilaterality is particularly common with paresthesia of the lips and tongue. Indeed, one may go so far as to say that if a reliable witness insists that his or her aura symptoms have never departed from one or the other side, the diagnosis of migraine must itself be regarded with some suspicion (see case 26).

Migrainous paresthesia may spread in two ways, either by direct extension to contiguous portions of the body surface (tactile field), or by the inauguration of new, separate foci elsewhere in the tactile field.

Other Sensory Hallucinations

Hallucinations of the other special senses are uncommon in migraine aura, although I should judge them to be notably commoner than most accounts allow for. Auditory hallucinations generally take the form of hissing, growling, or rumbling noises, which may be succeeded or preceded by dullness or loss of hearing. There may also be more highly organized hallucinations, especially of *music*, which may be "heard" with such vividness and verisimilitude that the patient immediately imagines there is a record or radio playing. Sometimes the same tune—usually a popular one—is heard in every migraine aura—precisely as occurs in "musical epilepsy" (see p. 165; and my article "Musical Ears," *London Review of Books* [3–16 May 1984]). Hallucinations of smell have been described to me by several patients: the smell is usually intense, unpleasing, strangely familiar yet unspecifiable, and often associated with forced reminiscence and feelings of *déjà vu*—symptoms reminiscent of those occurring in uncinate seizures. Hallucinations of taste are perhaps the least common of the special sense hallucinations.

A variety of visceral and epigastric symptoms may occur during migraine aura. The commonest, perhaps, is intense nausea of a quality which observant patients can distinguish from the subsequent nausea associated with headache, and other occurrences. Other patients describe a variety of sensation in the epigastrium— one patient of mine had a sensation of "vibrating wires" in the pit of the stomach (see case 19)—sensations which may rise through the chest toward the throat, often accompanied by eructation or forced swallowing.

Hallucinations of motion may take two forms. Rarely, there may occur what Gowers has termed a "motor sensation," for example, the feeling that a limb has moved, or the body has adopted a new posture, when in fact there has been no such movement. Far commoner, and perhaps the most intolerable of all aura symptoms, is intense sudden vertigo accompanied by staggering, overwhelming nausea and, frequently, vomiting. The following description is taken from Liveing, and relates, yet again, to the unfortunate "Mr. A" who appeared subject to every conceivable symptom of migraine:

His megrim seizures usually commence with blindness, and giddiness is only exceptional and slight. On one or two occasions, however, he has suffered from short attacks of intense vertigo, which have appeared to him to replace the ordinary fit. On waking one morning, before moving or rising in bed, he was alarmed to see all objects in the room revolving with extraordinary velocity from right to left in vertical circles . . . an almost exclusively visual vertigo. Lying perfectly still with closed eyes, the attack passed off in about the same time as that occupied by the blind period of his ordinary seizures.

Pseudo-objectivity of Migraine Hallucinations

We have used the term *hallucination* to denote the sensory experiences which may occur during a migraine aura, and the use of this word—which carries pejorative implications to many ears—must be justified. The hallmarks of the hallucinatory experience are these: it is mistaken for reality, and it elicits a perceptual reaction, in Konorski's term a *targeting reflex* (Konorski, 1967). Thus dreams are true hallucinations because they are experienced as reality, and associated with targeting reflexes of the eyes (the "rapid eye movements" of paradoxical sleep) as these scan the projected hallucinations. The abnormal sensations of a migraine aura, opposed to those of dreams, are likely to be experienced in full waking consciousness (although they may also occur in twilight states, or in sleep), and most patients learn not to mistake them for reality. Nevertheless there exists, even in the most sophisticated patients, a *tendency* to objectivize the sensations of the aura. Patients with paresthesia may look down at the affected hand or rub it. Patient 67, a highly intelligent physician who had experienced many auras with negative scotomata, would invariably feel that the illumination of the room was at fault, before realizing that she was experiencing a migraine aura. Many patients take off their spectacles and polish them carefully if they start to experience a migrainous shimmering. The sense of objectivity may be particularly striking where scintillating scotomata or olfactory hallucinations are experienced. Gowers (1904) remarks on the strength and stubbornness of this "involuntary sense of objectivity," and comments particularly on patients with pericentral scotomata who insist that they see a sort of angled crown or rainbow above the eyes (as drawn, by a patient, in *figure 2e*). Patient 75, a physician, who had had ample experience of the illusory nature of migraine auras, would always start searching for the cause of the smell when he experienced an olfactory aura. In the most severe auras, to be described below, the subjective sensations may completely overwhelm the patient and be experienced, like a dream, as total reality.

General Alterations of Sensory Threshold

A *diffuse* enhancement or obfuscation of sensation may occur in addition to, or in place of, the specific sensory hallucinations we have described. Such changes have already been alluded to in the context of common migraine, but may reach an exalted intensity in migraine aura.

Some patients describe an overall brightening of vision. In the words of one of my patients, a man who had never experienced scintillating scotomata: "It was as if a thousand-watt bulb had been turned on in the room." Further evidence of such diffuse visual excitation is provided by the intense, protracted, sometimes almost dazzling, visual after-images which may occur at such times, and the furor of brilliant visual images which are seen if the eyes are closed. Analogous phenomena may occur with respect to hearing, the faintest sounds appearing overwhelmingly loud, and being followed by protracted echoing or reverberation for some seconds after they have ceased. The faintest touch, similarly, may be exaggerated and intolerable. This state is thus one of an excruciating overall sensitivity, patients being *assaulted* by sensory stimuli from their environment, or by internal images and hallucinations if they insulate themselves from their environment. Such states are often succeeded by a relative, and on occasion, absolute extinction of sensation, especially in severe auras where syncope occurs. Such a course is reminiscent of the much more acute sensory extinction which may occur in epilepsy, as in a case of Gowers: ". . . for a moment all was silent, then all was dark, then consciousness was lost" (see case 19).

Alterations of Consciousness and Postural Tone

It seems probable that all migraine auras commence with some degree of *arousal,* whether this is manifested as multiform positive hallucinations, or states of analeptic excitement (as in case 67 and case 69). Such states of arousal may be difficult to distinguish from hyperactive migrainous prodromes, and sometimes present themselves as the climax of such states.

As the positive are succeeded by the negative hallucinations, so a generalized arousal of consciousness and muscular tonus—the hyperalert, tense, and vigilant phase—is succeeded by a waning of conscious level and tonus. In milder cases, this may be felt merely as a dullness and listlessness; in extreme cases there may be a total extinction of consciousness and/or an almost cataplectic loss of muscular tone.

Migrainous syncope is never of abrupt onset and offset, like a *petit mal* attack; the patient sinks into it over the course of a few minutes, and regains his faculties in the same gradual fashion. It is convenient to recognize three stages in this context: first, a state of torpor and lethargy; secondly, a state of stupor in which the patient may suffer "forced" thought and imagery, generally with an unpleasing quality—Liveing speaks of "horrid trances" at this stage, in which vivid forced imagery is allied to akinesia (a state reminiscent of narcolepsy or "sleep paralysis"); thirdly, a state of coma, which is likely to be accompanied by incontinence, and, very occasionally, by seizure-activity.

It is difficult to assess the overall incidence of migraine syncope, for it may occur only once or twice in a lifetime in a given patient, and the fact of its occurrence may have been forgotten or suppressed. Thus Lees and Watkins report the following case under the label of "basilar migraine":

A woman of 24 had had periodic attacks of bilateral visual disturbance, and numbness of the lips, tongue, and one arm, followed by frontal headache and faintness. . . . *Once*, at the height of the attack, she became unconscious, and was incontinent of urine and feces.

I myself have seen more than a hundred patients with migraine aura or classical migraine, and of these only four suffered syncopes with any regularity.

The incidence of *occasional* migraine syncopes may be very much higher. Thus, Selby and Lance found that "sixty patients (out of 396) had lost consciousness in association with attacks of headache," and that in eighteen of these sixty the impairment of consciousness was profound, and accompanied by features suggestive of an epileptic seizure.

Specific Motor Disorders

"Features suggestive of an epileptic seizure": these features, in the minds of most patients, are unconsciousness and convulsions.

We have discussed the incidence and quality of impaired or lost consciousness, as this occurs during migraine attacks, and we must now inquire whether true convulsions or spasms of epileptoid type may not also occur as a component of migraines. It is not denied that such motor symptoms, if their existence be accepted, are rare, far rarer than their epileptic counterparts; what we must question is the assertion, frequently and dogmatically made, that the higher disorders of migraine are exclusively sensory. Accounts of muscular *spasms* may be found in many of the classical writings on the subject, particularly those of Tissot, Liveing and Gowers:

A young girl of 12 years became suddenly ill with a violent migraine that occupied her eye, the temple and ear of the left side of the head; at the same time she had a tingling sensation as if of swarms of ants that began with the little finger on the same side, soon reaching the other fingers, the forearm, the arm, the neck, causing a violent retraction of the head by spasmodic movements. The spasm involved her lower jaw, accompanied by a general weakness of her entire body, without, however, losing consciousness. This cruel access was terminated by vomiting bilious water.

—Tissot, 1790

In one patient each attack of headache was preceded by sudden tingling in the calf, followed by painful cramp in the calf muscles, lasting a few minutes only. The same patient, however, had at other times attacks in which her face suddenly became crimson, sharp pains occurred in the head, and seemed to pass down the side to the leg, which was then 'drawn up' in spasm for a few minutes.

—Gowers, 1892

If such spasms occur, Gowers remarks, "the case usually diverges very much from the type, and sometimes is of such a character as to render it doubtful whether it should be classed with migraine or not."

A transient motor weakness in a limb (as opposed to the protracted hemiplegias which are discussed in the following chapter) is not uncommon, and may follow the passage of paresthesiae. In some such cases the apparent weakness resolves itself, on questioning or examining the patient, into an apractic rather than a paralytic deficit, but in other patients, of whom I have seen and examined a number during this stage of an aura, the limb may be toneless, without reflexes and truly paralyzed.

I have never witnessed a convulsion during a migraine aura, although I have been told by three patients (out of a total of 150 patients with classical migraine or isolated auras) that others had witnessed such convulsions during their attacks. The existence of such convulsions at the height of a migraine aura has been repeatedly attested by competent observers. Such accounts, indeed, may be traced into antiquity, the archetype of such attacks having been described by Aretaeus in the second century, a man in whom the appearance of a migraine spectrum was followed by loss of consciousness and convulsions.

How should we categorize such attacks? As atypical migraines with migrainous convulsions, as atypical epilepsies with migranoid features, or as attacks of epilepsy superimposed on migraines? Lennox neatly evades the dilemma by speaking of "hybrid seizures," and until we know more this is as good a term as any.

Addendum

G. W. Bruyn, who is a great authority on both chorea and migraines, has observed, on occasion, chorea *during* migraines. His observations opened my own eyes to what I had undoubtedly "seen" previously, but yet—overlooked. Since the first edition of *Migraine* I have seen, on at least a dozen occasions, the onset of complex motor excitements in migraine aura, with the appearance of chorea, and sometimes tics as well, set against a background of extreme motor restlessness, irritability, and drive (akathisia).

A special and specific significance is brought out by Bruyn, in relation to the basic mechanism(s) and pathogenesis of migraine. Chorea—a twinkling movement, or motor scintillation—does not have its origin in the cerebral cortex, but in the deeper parts of the brain, the basal ganglia and upper brainstem which are the parts that mediate normal awakening. Thus these observations of chorea during migraine support the notion that migraine is a sort of arousal-disorder, something located in the strange borderlands of sleep (see pp. 47–49, and chapter 5)—a disorder which has its origin deep in the brainstem, and not superficially, in the cortical mantle, as is often supposed (a matter further discussed in Part III of this book).

Alterations of Affect and Mood

We have described the profound mood disturbances which may precede and accompany successive stages of a common migraine or migraine equivalent. We must now consider symptoms altogether more acute, more dramatic, and different in quality from such mood changes, notably the sudden eruptions of overwhelming "forced" affect which may occur in the course of severe migraine auras.

Like migrainous syncope, this is a relatively uncommon symptom, and rarely occurs with consistency in every attack the patient experiences; nevertheless, most patients with severe frequent auras have occasionally experienced such sudden eruptions of affect. Thus one patient (case 11), whose history is later detailed, who had had attacks of classical migraine or isolated aura since childhood which inconvenienced but rarely discomposed her, experienced on one occasion "a perfectly frightful sense of foreboding" during the course of an aura. She herself recognized that this was an exceptional feature of some of her attacks, and in no sense a mere anxious expectation of a banal sequence with which she was entirely familiar, and to which she was wholly inured.

Such states of sudden overwhelming affect have been richly documented in the earlier literature, especially by Liveing (with respect to migraine attacks) and by Gowers (on epilepsy). Thus Liveing observed that there were sufferers "who cannot bear to think or talk of their attacks, and always refer to them with horror, which is clearly not on account of the pain they occasion." Gowers observed in connection with epilepsy that the emotional aura usually took the form of *fear* ("vague alarm or intense terror") although he provides case histories of other types of affect being experienced. The most acute form of such fear may reach appalling intensity, and convey to the patient a sense of imminent destruction or death. This sense of mortal fear (which may also occur in association with attacks of angina, pulmonary embolism, etc.) was called by the older physicians "angor animi," a term which cannot be bettered. The affective reaction is not always in this direction. A few patients may experience a sense of mild *pleasure* or delight in the course of their auras (see case 16), and on rare occasions this may be exalted toward states of profound *awe* or *rapture* (see appendix to this chapter).

Again the affect, though intense, may lack the gravity of dread or rapture, and convey only a sense of fun or *hilarity* to the patient, or "silliness" to an observer (see case 65): Selby and Lance refer, rather curtly, to "apparently hysterical behavior" in such cases.

Gowers records, in one epileptic patient, an access of pure moral feeling ("whatever was taking place before the patient would suddenly appear to be *wrong*—i.e., morally wrong") immediately prior to loss of consciousness and convulsion. A complex feeling which may also present itself with great force and suddenness, in these auras, is a feeling of *absurdity*. One of the commonest of these abrupt feeling-states (it cannot be called purely affective) is the sense of sudden *strangeness,* which may occur as an isolated feeling, or as an accompaniment of some of the affective states we have discussed: the sense of strangeness is frequently accompanied by a sense of profoundly disturbed time-perception.

In summary, we may recognize the following features as characteristic of these states in migraine auras:

(1) Their sudden onset.
(2) Their apparent sourcelessness, and frequent incongruity with the foreground contents of consciousness.
(3) Their overwhelming quality.
(4) A sense of passivity, and of the affect being "forced" into the mind.
(5) Their brief duration (they rarely last more than a few minutes).
(6) The sense of stillness and timelessness they convey: such states may wax in depth or intensity, but this occurs despite the absence of any experimental "happening."
(7) Their difficulty or impossibility of adequate description.

Such states of overwhelming "forced" feeling may occur not only in cerebral paroxysms as migraine and epilepsy, but in schizophrenic and drug-induced psychoses, in feverish and toxic states, in hysterical, ecstatic, and dream states. We are inevitably reminded of William James' listing of the qualities of "mystical" states: ineffability, abstract quality, transiency, passivity.

Alterations of Highest Integrative Function

It has been held by a number of eminent clinical observers that the cerebral disorders of migraine occur only at primitive levels, and that the existence of subtler disorders, should they occur, is indicative of epilepsy or of some organic pathology. This view is erroneous. An immense number of complex cerebral symptoms may occur in the context of indisputable migraines, symptoms fully as numerous and diverse as their epileptic counterparts.

One might, indeed, suspect that alterations of higher cerebral function occur in the majority of migraine auras, but may escape notice through their subtlety or strangeness, or because the patient was not undertaking any intricate intellectual or motor activity at the time of the aura. Thus, Alvarez, a careful witness of his own migraines, has described how he became aware, one day, that his auras were not merely "pure," isolated visual phenomena:

Often, when fuzzy-eyed and unable to read comfortably, I have employed my time writing a family letter, longhand. Later, on checking the letter, I had written words other than the ones I had thought I was writing.

It is easily understood how a subtle dyslexic or dysphasic deficit of this type may fail to be noticed by a majority of patients. Leading questions will often be required to elicit the exact nature of such symptoms. Many patients may confess that they feel "strange" or "confused" during a migraine aura, that they are clumsy in their movements, or that they would not drive at such a time. In short, they may be aware of *something* the matter in addition to the scintillating scotoma, paresthesia, and other occurrences, something so unprecedented in their experience, so difficult to describe, that it is often avoided or omitted when speaking of their complaints. Great patience and minute exactitude are needed to define the subtler symptoms of migraine aura, and only if these are employed will the frequency and importance of such symptoms be realized.

It may be stated that the more complex disorders of the cerebral function usually occur *after* the simpler phenomena (although this is not invariably so), and it may be possible to obtain descriptions of elaborate sequences: thus the simplest visual manifestations—

dots, lines, stars, and so forth—may be succeeded by a scintillating scotoma, and this in turn by bizarre alterations of perception (zoom vision, mosaic vision, etc.), finally culminating in elaborate illusory images or dreamlike states. We may recognize the following important categories of disturbance:

(a) Complex disorders of visual perception (conveniently described as Lilliputian, Brobdingnagian, zoom, mosaic, cinematographic vision, etc.)

(b) Complex difficulties in the perception and use of the body (apraxic and agnosic symptoms).

(c) The entire gamut of speech and language disorders.

(d) States of double or multiple consciousness, often associated with feelings of *déjà vu* or *jamais vu*, and other disorders and dislocations of time-perception.

(e) Elaborate dreamy, nightmarish, trancelike, or delirious states.

These categories are isolated for convenience only, and, far from being mutually exclusive, they overlap at many levels; many or all of these disorders may occur simultaneously in the course of a severe migraine aura. We may first describe some of these symptoms in greater detail, and then proceed to the presentation of illustrative case histories.

Lilliputian vision (micropsia) denotes an apparent diminution, and *Brobdingnagian vision* (macropsia) an apparent enlargement, in the size of objects, although the terms may also be used to denote the apparent approach or recession of the visual world—these representing alternative descriptions or hallucinations or disordered size: distance constancy. If such changes occur gradually rather than abruptly, the patient will experience *zoom vision*—an opening-out, or closing-down, in the size of objects as if observing them through the changing focal lengths of a "zoom" lens. The most famous descriptions of such perceptual changes have, of course, been provided by Lewis Carroll, who was himself subject to dramatic classical migraines of this type. A scintillating scotoma itself has no external location, and may therefore be projected as an "artifact" of any size, at any distance (see case 69).

Mosaic and Cinematic Vision

The term *mosaic vision* denotes the fracture of the visual image into irregular, crystalline, polygonal facets, dovetailed together as in a mosaic. The size of the facets tends to pass through an evolution from small to large, and then back again. When they are extremely fine, the visual world presents an appearance of crystalline iridescence or "graininess," reminiscent of a pointilliste painting (shown schematically in *figure 4b*). As the facets become larger, the visual image takes on the appearance of a classical mosaic (*figure 4c*), and with their increasing enlargement a "cubist" appearance. Finally, when the component facets come to compete in size with the total visual image, the latter becomes impossible to recognize (*figure 4d*), and a peculiar form of visual agnosia is experienced.

The term *cinematographic vision* denotes the nature of visual experience when the illusion of motion has been lost. At such times, the patient sees only a rapidly flickering series of "stills," as in a film run too slowly. The rate of flickering is of the same order as the scintillation-rate of migrainous scotomata or paresthesia (six to twelve per second), but may accelerate during the course of the aura to restore the appearance of normal motion, or (in a particularly severe, delirious aura) the appearance of a continuously modulated visual hallucination.*

Both of these rare symptoms have been recorded as occurring in the course of epileptic seizures, and, more commonly, during acute psychoses, whether drug-induced or schizophrenic. The famous cat-painter Louis Wain experienced a variety of visual misperceptions during phases of acute schizophrenic psychosis, including mosaic vision, and was able to provide remarkable records of the experiences (*figure 5*).

Addendum

When I originally wrote *Migraine,* I considered the phenomena of "mosaic" and "cinematic" vision of extreme importance. They show

---

*An extremely detailed personal account of mosaic and cinematic vision, as experienced in a severe attack of migraine, is given in my book *A Leg to Stand On* (New York: Summit Books, 1984), pp. 95–101.

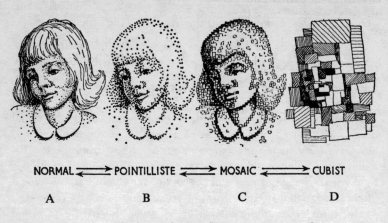

NORMAL ⇌ POINTILLISTE ⇌ MOSAIC ⇌ CUBIST

A   B   C   D

Figure 4. The stages of "mosaic" vision, as experienced
during migraine aura (see text)

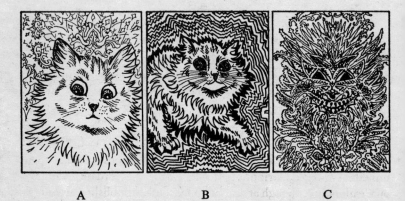

A   B   C

Figure 5. Some visual hallucination in acute psychosis

These drawings of cats, depicted by a schizophrenic artist (Louis Wain) during a very
acute psychosis, formalize certain perceptual alterations which may also occur during
migraine aura. In *figure 5a*, the face is set upon a background of swarming brilliant
starlike figures: in *figure 5b*, concentric shimmering waves expand from the point
of fixation: in *figure 5c*, the entire image has been transformed to a mosaic pattern.

us how the brain-mind constructs "space" and "time," by demonstrating to us what happens when space and time are broken, or *unmade*.

In a scotoma, as we have observed, the idea of space itself is extinguished along with the extinction of the visual field, and we are left with "no trace, space, or place." In mosaic and cinematic vision we seem to be presented with an intermediary state which has an inorganic, crystalline character, but no organic personal character, no "life."

This too, like scotomata may inspire a strange horror.

Other Disturbances

Many other forms of visual misperception have been described in migraine auras. Objects may appear to have unnaturally sharp contours, to be diagrammatic, to be flattened and without a third dimension, to be set in an exaggerated perspective, and so on.

A particularly detailed description of complex visual hallucinations in migraine has been provided by Klee (1968) who describes many forms of *metamorphopsia* occurring during migraine auras: distortion of contours, monocular diplopias, reduced discrimination of contrast (leading, on occasion, to effective blindness), waviness of linear components in visual images and formation of concentric haloes (compare Louis Wain's drawings above), and others. He also records examples of color changes in visual images, and eccentric misplacements within the visual field other than micropsia and macropsia. Classical scotomata, positive and negative, are relatively infrequent in Klee's series. Both simple and complex visual hallucinations, Klee observes, are much more commonly diffuse than unilateral in their distribution; this finding is in accordance with my own experience, though at odds with most other published accounts. Occasionally a patient may suffer from *simultagnosia*—an inability to recognize more than one object at a time, and thus to construct a complex visual picture.*

---

*I have recently seen a patient who gives an extremely clear description of such a visual agnosia following a scintillating scotoma. In this state he finds it very difficult, for example, to tell the time from looking at his watch. He must first gaze at one

Analogous phenomena may occur with reference to body image and body movements. Sometimes (especially after the passage of intense paresthesia in a limb) a portion of the body may feel magnified, diminished, distorted, or absent. It may be impossible to examine or perceive adequately the nature of an object held in the hand (one cannot clearly distinguish the sensory from the motor components in such cases, for sensation is always active and exploratory; one should perhaps speak of *apractagnosia* in this context). Higher sensory and motor deficits of this type are often mistaken for elementary anesthesias and paralyses. One must consider separately difficulties in planning complex sensory-motor tasks; Pribram has called these *scotomata of action*. These are of great practical importance, and may underlie, for example, the patient's discovery that he cannot drive a car or organize a long sentence or a complex sequence of actions, during the course of a migraine aura.

Speech difficulties of this type have been termed (by Luria) *dynamic aphasias*. Other types of aphasia may also occur in the course of a migraine aura. The commonest of these is the occurrence of an expressive aphasia, which may be associated with bilateral paresthesia of the lips and tongue, and apractic difficulties using the oral and vocal muscles. Occurring sometimes in the wake of auditory misperception or hallucination, there may occur a sensory aphasia,

---

hand, then at the other, then at all the figures in turn, and in this way, very slowly and laboriously, he will "puzzle out" the time. If he just glances at his watch-face, as he would normally do, it appears absolutely unintelligible to him. In effect the watch has lost its physiognomy—its "face." It can no longer be perceived as an organic whole, synthetically, but has to be broken down, analyzed, feature by feature, part by part. Such a loss of qualitative or "synthetic" perception may occur rather commonly, and disconcertingly, in migraine. A particularly striking and disconcerting form of this disorder is the sudden inability to recognize a *face,* to see it as familiar, as a whole, indeed *as* a face. This singular (and frightening and sometimes comic) disorder is termed *prosopagnosia.* (I have described this disorder in detail in an article, "The Man Who Mistook His Wife for a Hat," *London Review of Books* 5, no. 9 [May 1983].) Similar breakdowns in synthetic perception may also occur in the sphere of audition. *Voices* may lose their characteristic quality, become inexpressive and toneless, completely unvoicelike. Music similarly may lose its tonality and musical character, becoming an unintelligible mere noise, during a migrainous *amusia* aura. At such time, the very *idea* of music is lost (as in prosopagnosia the very *idea* of faces is lost); and in our patient bewildered before his watch, the very *idea* of a time-telling watch face.

in which speech sounds like "noise," and the perception of its phonemic structure is lost.*

Among the strangest and most intense symptoms of migraine aura, and the most difficult of description or analysis, are the occurrence of feelings of sudden familiarity and certitude (*déjà vu*), or its opposite, feelings of sudden strangeness and unfamiliarity (*jamais vu*). Such states are experienced, momentarily and occasionally, by everyone; their occurrence in migraine auras (as in epileptic auras, psychoses, etc.) is marked by their overwhelming intensity and relatively long duration. These states are necessarily associated with a multitude of other feelings: the thought that time has stopped, or is mysteriously recapitulating itself; the feeling that one is dreaming, or momentarily transported to another world; feelings of intense nostalgia, in *déjà vu*, sometimes associated with an uprush of long-forgotten memories; feelings of clairvoyance, in *déjà vu;* or of the world or oneself being newly minted, in *jamais vu;* and in all cases, the feeling that consciousness has been doubled.

There is (1) the quasi-parasitical state of consciousness (dreamy state), and (2) there are remains of normal consciousness and thus, there is double consciousness . . . a mental diplopia.

Thus Hughlings Jackson describes the doubling of consciousness.** No description is ever adequate for the elaborate yet unmis-

---

*We are describing certain sensory, motor, and conceptual symptoms of migraine aura in their severest forms, in order to clarify the type of cerebral disturbance which is involved. Frequently, however, such symptoms may present themselves as no more than a very mild disturbance, in particular as a tendency toward *mistakes* of various kinds: mishearing, mislaying, misreading words, slips of the tongue, slight lapses of memory, and similar occurrences. Freud, himself a sufferer from classical migraines, comments on such errors: "Slips of tongue do indeed occur most frequently when one is tired, or has a headache, or feels an attack of migraine coming on. Forgetting proper names very often occurs in these circumstances; many people are habitually warned of the onset of an attack of migraine by the inability to recall proper names" (1920).

**A variety of psychological and physiological theories have been advanced to explain *déjà vu* and the symptoms with which it is commonly linked. Thus Freud ascribes the uncanniness of the experience to a sudden return of repressed material, while Efron sees *déjà vu*, aphasia, and subjective time distortions—when linked together—as representing an alteration of "time labelling" in the nervous system. These two theories are in different dimensions of explanation, and are perfectly compatible with one another.

takable sensation of *déjà vu* and all that goes with it, and the most vivid descriptions are found outside medical literature:

We have all some experience of a feeling which comes over us occasionally, of what we are saying and doing, having been said or done before, in a remote time—of our having been surrounded, dim ages ago, by the same faces, objects, and circumstances—of our knowing perfectly what will be said next, as if we suddenly remembered it.

—Dickens: *David Copperfield*

> Moreover, something is or seems
> That touches me with mystic gleams,
> Like glimpses of forgotten dreams—
>
> Of something felt, like something here;
> Of something done, I know not where;
> Such as no language may declare.

—Tennyson: *The Two Voices*

One of the wonders of opium is to transform instantaneously an unknown room into a room so familiar, so full of memories, that one thinks one has always occupied it.

—Cocteau: *Opium**

The terms *"dreamy state"* and *"delirium"* require some clarification in the context of migraine auras. One type of dreamy state is that associated with *déjà vu* and doubling of consciousness; in such cases there may be "forced reminiscence," or the unfolding of a stereotyped, unchanging, reiterative dream sequence or memory

---

*A number of people, learning that forced reminiscence and *déjà vu* experiences are particularly common in epilepsy, migraine, psychosis, and so forth, become alarmed for their own health or sanity. They may be reassured in the words of Hughlings Jackson: "I should never . . . [he writes] diagnose epilepsy from the paroxysmal occurrence of reminiscence without other symptoms, although I should suspect epilepsy, if that super-positive mental state began to occur very frequently . . . I have never been consulted for 'reminiscence' only; there have always been in the cases I have seen, at the time I have seen them, with this and other forms of 'dreamy state,' ordinary, although often very slight, symptoms of epilepsy."

Such states of dreamy reminiscence are quite frequent in classical migraines. The most detailed accounts of them have been given to me, however, in the context of epilepsy (see "Musical Ears," *London Review of Books*, May 1984).

sequence in every attack. Such sequences are perhaps commoner in (psychomotor) epilepsy than in migraine, but they undoubtedly occur in the latter. Penfield and Perot (1963), who have investigated these phenomena in remarkable detail, and have succeeded in eliciting such reiterative sequences by the stimulation of certain cortical points, regard them as "fossilized" dream-sequences preserved as such in the cortex, precise replicas of past experience; they appear to be mnemonic images which unfold, given the initial activation (epileptic, migrainous, experimental, etc.) at the same rate as the initial perceptual experience.

Different from these stereotyped, reiterative sequences, but with something of the same coercive quality, are freewheeling states of hallucinosis, illusion or "dreaming" which may be experienced during intense migraine auras, and be manifest as confused or confabulatory states of which the patient retains imperfect recollection. These states are composed of coherent, dramatically organized series of images, and are usually compared by patients to intense, involuntary day-dreams or daymares (see cases 72 and 19).

It is impossible to make a clear dividing line between these "dreamy states" and migrainous deliria or psychoses. The degree of disorganization in a delirium is greater, and the patient may experience only an effervescence of elementary sensations (dots, stars, lattices, tessellated forms,* tinnitus, buzzing, formication, etc.), which have not been elaborated to the level of concrete images. In profound migraine deliria, the patient presents a muttering, restless (twitching or tossing) picture strongly reminiscent of a febrile delirium or delirium tremens. Gowers (1907) observes that migraine

---

*A vivid account of tessellated hallucinations is provided in Klee's monograph, one of his patients experiencing, on one occasion, a vision of red and green triangles moving towards her, on other occasions hexagonal black figures surrounding a shining circle, and on many occasions a shimmering of red and yellow, which looked like a waving, checked blanket.

In a fascinating article based partly on his own experiences ("The Fortification Illusions of Migraine" *Scientific American* 224, 5 [May 1971] 88–96), Dr. W. Richards describes repeating hexagonal motifs as a highly characteristic feature of migraine hallucinations and speculates that this reflects the functional organization of the visual cortex in hexagonal units. Repeating geometrical and especially hexagonal patterns have been reported in almost all forms of primitive visual hallucinations, and are regarded by Klüver as "hallucinatory constants."

is "often attended by quiet delirium of which nothing can be subsequently recalled," and describes one such patient who at the
height of her attack "passed into a delirious state, making strange
statements, of which she afterwards remembered nothing. Her condition was described by a doctor who saw her as resembling epileptic
mania."*

The swarming figments of delirium are occasionally organized
into a multitude of minute (Lilliputian) hallucinations, as in the
following case history provided by Klee (1968):

The patient . . . was a 38-year-old man who suffered from attacks of severe
migraine associated with subacute delirious state and delirium. As a rule
he had amnesia for the greater part of the time during which the attacks
lasted. During his admission he was, however, able to report that during
his attacks he had on one occasion seen 20 cm high, greyish-colored Red
Indians crowding round in the room in which he lay. He was not afraid of
them, as they did not seem to have anything to do with him. On another
occasion he lay and picked up hallucinatory musical instruments from the
floor.**

---

*Some clarification of this complex twilight zone in which "delirium," "mania,"
"dreamy states," and "confusion" have been reported is perhaps afforded by the very
recent recognition that so-called transient global amnesia (TGA) may occur with
significant frequency in classical migraine attacks. Indeed, it has been suggested
that this spectacular syndrome—in which the patient may not only lose all short-
term memory but may develop a profound retrograde amnesia—may be chiefly or
exclusively migrainous in nature. In such an amnesia the patient may not only lose
the ability to recognize family friends, people, and places from the present but may
after recovery have no recollection of headache, nausea, scotomata, etc., of which
they complained when in the throes of the attack. (G. F. Crowell et al., *Archives of
Neurology* 41 [1984] 75–79). I have written at length about the almost incredible
effects of profound retrograde amnesia in "The Lost Mariner," *New York Review of
Books* (February 1984).

**Lilliputian hallucinations are notoriously associated with alcoholic deliria, and,
less commonly, with intoxication by ether, cocaine, hashish, or opium—Theophile
Gautier has provided delightful descriptions of such hallucinatory, drug-induced
elves. Myriads of minute hallucinations may occur in the excitements of general
paresis (Baudelaire). Sufferers from feverish deliria may experience Lilliputian hallucinations, as described by de Musset. Fasting, inanition, and infected flagellations
may have played a part in causing the minute hallucinations of certain mystics
(e.g., Joan of Arc). Leroy (1922), reviewing the subject, observes that whereas
"ordinary toxic visions may produce a feeling of fear and terror, Lilliputian visions
are accompanied, on the contrary, by a feeling of curiosity and amusement."

Very rarely, the profound delirium of a migraine aura may last throughout the ensuing (classical) migraine, and in such cases—as with all extended deliria—may be structured into the form of an acute hallucinatory psychosis. Mingazzini (1926) provided classical descriptions of such states (*hemikranischen Psykosen*) and a particularly vivid case history has recently been provided by Klee (1968):

During a particularly severe attack which lasted for a week, the patient became psychotic and it was necessary to admit her to a mental hospital. The patient had amnesia for the episode. . . . It appears that during the day preceding her admission she had been increasingly restless with clouding of consciousness, she had heard her neighbors making unpleasant comments about her, and also she believed that she had been stuck with knives. During the first days of her admission she was disoriented, restless, and presumably hallucinated in both hearing and sight: she heard children's voices and the voice of her general practitioner, she believed that her legs had been amputated, and that people were shooting at her through the window. This psychotic episode disappeared within a few days. . . .

It must be emphasized that a migrainous psychosis of this magnitude is exceedingly rarely seen. Klee, in his unique series of 150 patients with migraine severe enough to warrant hospital admission, observed recurrent migraine psychoses in only two of these. I have seen only a single such case myself, in a patient who was schizophrenic: his acute psychoses, however, occurred only in the context of intense classical migraines.

Transient states of *depersonalization* are appreciably commoner during migraine auras. Freud reminds us that "the ego is first and foremost a body-ego . . . the mental projection of the surface of the body." The sense of "self" appears to be based, fundamentally, on a continuous inference from the stability of body image, the stability of outward perceptions, and the stability of time perception. Feelings of ego dissolution readily and promptly occur if there is serious disorder or instability of body image, external perception, or time-perception, and all of these, as we have seen, may occur during the course of a migraine aura.

Case Histories

The following three case histories are taken from Liveing's monograph, and are presented *in extenso* in view of their clarity and graphic power.

Forced reminiscence, time-distortion, and doubled consciousness
As the visual phenomena passed off, he experienced a singular disorder of ideation; circumstances and events which had occurred long before were brought back to him as if actually present; his consciousness appeared to be doubled, and the past and the present confounded.

Forced thinking, confusion, and multiple dysphasic symptoms
For about half an hour, one series of ideas forced themselves involuntarily on my mind. I could not free myself from the strange ideas which existed in my head. I endeavored to speak . . . but found that I spoke uniformly other words than those intended. . . . It became necessary that I should write a receipt for some money that I had received on account of the poor. I seated myself and wrote the first two words, but in a moment found that I was incapable of proceeding, for I could not recollect the words which belonged to the ideas which were present in my mind. . . . I tried to write one letter slowly after the others . . . but remarked that the characters I was writing were not those which I wished to write. . . . For about half an hour there reigned a kind of tumultuary disorder in my senses. . . . I endeavored, as much as lay in my power, considering the great crowd of confused images which presented themselves to my mind, to recall my principles of religion, of conscience, of future expectation. . . . Thank God, this state did not continue very long, for in about half an hour my head began to grow clearer, the strange and tiresome ideas became less vivid and turbulent. . . . At last, I found myself as clear and serene as in the beginning of the day. *All that remained now was a slight headache*.

When migraine auras reach their ultimate intensity, the "great crowd of confused images," of which the above patient speaks, assume hallucinatory form, and blot out the world around him. Jones has reminded us that "attacks in every way indistinguishable from the classical nightmare may not only occur but may run their whole course during the waking state," and such "daymares"—as they have been called—in their quality (feelings of dread, horror, paralysis) and duration (a few minutes) bear a remarkable similarity to delirious migraine auras. This clinical affinity does not, of course, imply that similar physiological mechanisms are necessarily involved.

Delirious migraine aura
He had been somewhat overworked at school, and on returning home early one day, was suddenly seized with what he called a 'day nightmare'. He

lost all conscious perception of the room and objects about him, and he felt himself hanging on the brink of a precipice, and other horrors which he could not remember or describe. His relatives were alarmed by hearing him cry out, and found him on the stairs in a kind of somnambulistic state, vociferating loudly. He recovered himself in about ten minutes, but remained a good deal shaken and distressed. . . . The second attack was of much the same kind, but occurred shortly after going to bed at night. . . . It was shortly after these attacks . . . that his megrim became fully established.

I shall pass now to a number of illustrative case histories taken from my own records.

Case 72

Dreamy state

This 44-year-old man had suffered from very occasional classical migraines since adolescence. His attacks would be ushered in by scintillating scotomata. In one attack, a profound dreamlike state followed the visual phenomena. He has described this as follows:

A very strange thing happened, shortly after my vision came back. First I couldn't think where I was, and then I suddenly realized that I was back in California. . . . It was a hot summer day. I saw my wife moving about on the veranda, and I called to her to bring me a Coke. She turned to me with an odd look on her face, and said: "Are you sick or something?" I suddenly seemed to wake up, and realized that it was a winter's day in New York, that there was no veranda, and that it wasn't my wife but my secretary who was standing in the office looking strangely at me.

Case 19

Scotomata, paresthesia, visceral aura and forced affect; occasional delirious auras; occasional aura "status"

This patient was a young man of 16 who had been prone to classical migraines and isolated auras since childhood. He has attacks with many different formats.

Most commonly they start with paresthesia in the left foot, rising toward the thigh. When these have reached the knee, a second focus of paresthesia starts in the right hand. As the paresthesia die away, there occurs a curious distortion of hearing, in which there appears to be a roaring sound in the ears, as if they were cupped by shells. Following this, he tends to get bilateral scintillating scotomata confined to the lower halves of both visual fields. . . .

On a few occasions, this patient has suffered from an aura 'status' lasting as much as five hours, constituted of alternating paresthesia in the feet, hands, and face.

On other occasions, the aura has started with a sensation of "tingling—like vibrating wires" in the epigastrium, associated with an intense sense of foreboding.

Yet other attacks, usually nocturnal, have a nightmarish quality. The initial symptoms are of compulsion and restlessness—"I feel edgy—like I got to get up and do something." Subsequently there develops a profound hallucinatory state: vertiginous hallucinations, hallucinations of being trapped in a speeding car, or of seeing heavy figures made of metal advancing upon him. As he emerges from this delirious state, he becomes conscious of paresthesiae and sometimes scotomata. These delirious aura are usually succeeded by intense headache.

This patient has also suffered a number of syncopal attacks in severe aura, in which the positive hallucinations have been followed by a simultaneous "fading" away of sight and hearing, a sense of faintness, and then unconsciousness.

Case 11

Classical migraine; loss of headache component in pregnancy; scintillating scotomata and negative scotomata; photogenic attacks; occasional "angor animi"

This patient was an extremely self-possessed and intelligent woman who had suffered from attacks of classical migraine, six to ten attacks yearly, except during pregnancy—when she had only isolated auras, and occasional periods of up to two years, when she had abdominal instead of cephalgic migraines.

The attacks were almost always ushered in by scintillating scotomata in either or both half-fields. The period of scintillation was found to be associated, if the patient closed her eyes, by exaggerated visual after-images and tumultuous visual imagery. Flickering light of certain frequencies would invariably elicit a scintillating scotoma. The visual aura would be followed by a "thrilling" sensation in the nose and tongue, and occasionally the hands. On a few occasions this patient experienced a "perfectly frightful sense of foreboding" during the aura. Negative scotomata were rare, always invested with intensely unpleasant affect, and invariably followed by a particularly severe headache.

Case 16

Visual aura; forced thinking and reminiscence; pleasurable affect; protracted sensory prodrome

A 55-year-old man with onset of classical migraine and isolated auras in childhood. He describes his auras with a certain fervor. "There is greater depth and speed and acuity of thought," he maintains. "I keep recalling things long forgotten, visions of earlier years will spring to my mind." He enjoys his auras, provided they are not succeeded by a migraine headache. His wife, however, is less impressed with them; she remarks that during his auras her husband "walks back and forth, talks in a repetitive manner in a sort of monotone; he seems to be in a trance, and is quite unlike his usual self."

This patient has consistently observed "luminous spots" fleeting across his visual fields for two to three days before each attack, and this visual excitation may be accompanied by prodromal excitement and euphoria.

Case 65

Aphasic and paresthetic aura accompanied by "silly" affect and forced laughter

This patient was a normally self-possessed girl of 15 subject to infrequent classical migraines of great severity. For a period of forty-five minutes, in my consulting room, she experienced an aura during which she giggled without intermission. During this time she was severely aphasic, and had paresthesiae flitting from one limb to another. When she recovered from this state, she apologized in these terms: "I don't know what I was laughing at—I just couldn't help it—everything seemed so funny, like laughing gas."

Case 69

Complex visual aura, preceded by intense arousal

A 23-year-old man with attacks of classical migraine and isolated aura since early adolescence. The onset of the attacks is heralded by hyperactivity and elation of almost maniacal intensity. Thus, on one morning, the patient—normally a sober motorcyclist—found himself driven to speed wildly, and to shout and sing while he did this. This was followed by a scintillating scotoma, accompanied by perceptual changes of higher order. He describes the concentric lines of the scotoma as like "the furrows in a ploughed field. . . . I could see them between the lines of the book I was reading, but the book looked huge, and the furrows seemed like great chasms, hundreds of feet behind the lines of print." As the scintillations died away, he experienced a "let-down, empty feeling, like after taking benzedrine."

On this occasion, the patient experienced a typical vascular headache and intense abdominal pain for the ensuing ten hours. These symptoms finally passed away, rather suddenly, and were succeeded by "a marvellous calm feeling."

Case 70

Mosaic and cinematographic vision

A 45-year-old man who had experienced frequent migraine auras and occasional classical migraines since childhood. The aura generally took the form of scintillating scotomata and paresthesia, but on a number of occasions he had experienced mosaic vision as a chief symptom. During these episodes he has observed that portions of the visual image, in particular faces, may appear "cut-up," distorted and disjointed, being composed of sharp-edged fragments. He compares this appearance to that of an early Picasso. More frequently he has experienced cinematographic vision, this type of aura being particularly prone to be evoked by flickering light of certain frequencies, for example, if his television set is improperly adjusted. The cinematographic vision may also be elicited, experimentally, by the flickering illumination of a "strobe" lamp. In either case, it will continue for several minutes following cessation of the provocative stimulus, and is generally followed by a severe classical migraine.*

Case 14

Multiple aura equivalents

A 48-year-old woman who suffered from classical migraines until the age of 20, but has had only isolated auras and migraine equivalents since this time. She has frequent attacks of scintillating scotomata unaccompanied by paresthesia, and occasional attacks of paresthesia, in the lips and hands, unaccompanied by scotomata. Severe scotomatous auras are accompanied by intense "angor animi," and are followed by syncope. She has, however, also suffered from syncopes of slow onset and offset, and also from attacks

---

*The restriction of mosaic vision to faces, in this patient and in others whom I have seen, suggests that the perception of faces *qua* faces must have a distinct and specific perceptual substrate. Certain other facts support such a view, notably the ability of infants to recognize faces before simple geometric shapes, and the occasional occurrence of a *prosopagnosia*—a specific inability to recognize faces—after certain cortical lesions. (See also footnote on pp. 87–88.)

of intense angst, unaccompanied by sensory hallucinations, and lasting ten to twenty minutes. All these appear to be variants of migraine aura.

Further varieties of migraine aura, as experienced at different times by the same individual, are quoted below through the courtesy of a colleague, who has suffered from frequent migraine auras, and occasional classical migraines, since childhood. He has provided short notes on a number of his attacks, and an elaborate description of two unusual attacks.

Case 75

(a) Nightmare, followed by sudden appearance of two white lights, blinking, drawing nearer with a jerking motion. Affect of intense terror, with feeling of incongruity with nightmare contents. Subsequent evolution of classical migraine.
(b) Nightmare, suddenly changing to cinematographic vision of flickering stills persisting for ten minutes in waking state.
(c) "Daymare" intruding on waking consciousness, with great anxiety, forced reminiscence, and dysphasia on attempting to speak. Duration about thirty minutes: no sequel.

The following description is quoted *in extenso:*

It was a late summer afternoon, and I was winding along a country road on my motorbike. An extraordinary sense of stillness came upon me, a feeling that I had lived this moment before, in the same place—although I had never travelled on this road before. I felt that this summer afternoon had always existed, and that I was arrested in an endless moment. When I got off the bike, a few minutes later, I had an extraordinarily powerful tingling in my hands, nose, lips and tongue. It seemed to be a continuation of the vibration of the motorbike, and at first I took this to be some simple after-effect. But no such explanation was tenable, for the vibrating sensation was growing stronger every moment, and appeared to be spreading, very slowly, from my fingertips to the palms of my hands, and then upwards. My sense of vision was then affected; a feeling of motion was communicated to everything I saw, so that the trees, the grass, the clouds, etc., seemed to exhibit a silent boiling, to be quivering and streaming upwards in a sort of ecstasy. The hum of crickets was all around me, and when I closed my eyes, this was immediately translated into a hum of color, which seemed to be the exact visual translation of the sound I heard. After about twenty minutes, the paresthesia, which had ascended to my elbows, retraced their course and disappeared, the visual world resumed its normal appearance, and the sense of ecstasy faded. I had a 'come-down' feeling, and the beginnings of a headache.

There are many points of interest in this detailed description; the elicitation of Jacksonian paresthesia apparently in resonance with the oscillation of the motorbike, a phenomenon which appears analogous to the elicitation of a scintillating scotoma by flickering light of the same frequency, the "boiling" motion of visual images, the sense of timelessness and *déjà vu,* and not least the experience of a synesthetic equivalence between auditory stimuli and visual images.

The following account is also quoted at length, because it conveys the typical quality of a migrainous delirium:

It started with the wallpaper, which I suddenly observed to be shimmering like the surface of water when agitated. A few minutes later, this was accompanied by a vibration in the right hand, as if it were resting on the sounding board of a piano. Then dots, flashes, moving slowly across the field of vision. Patterns, as of Turkish carpets, suddenly changing. Images of flowers continuously raying and opening out. Everything faceted and multiplied: bubbles rising toward me, apertures opening and closing honeycombs. These images are dazzling when I close my eyes, but still visible, more faintly, when the eyes are opened. They lasted twenty or thirty minutes, and were succeeded by a splitting headache.

Structure of the Aura

Migraines are often described, and misunderstood, because they are thought of in terms of a single symptom. Thus, a common migraine may be equated with a headache, and a migraine aura with a scotoma: such descriptions are ludicrously inadequate in a clinical sense, and permit the formulation of equally absurd physiological theories. The discussion and case histories presented in this chapter indicate the richness and complexity of aura symptoms. It is as rare to encounter a single symptom in the course of a migraine aura, as in a common migraine. Careful interrogation and observation will usually reveal that two, five, or a dozen manifestations are proceeding in unison. Nor are all of these manifestations likely to be on the same functional level (in the sense that scotomata and paresthesia may be presumed to be): simple circumscribed hallucinations projected on to the visual or tactile field are likely to be accompanied by sensory alterations of greater complexity (e.g., mosaic vision), disorders of arousal mechanisms (conscious level, etc.), of affect, and of highest integrative function.

Further, the symptoms of migraine aura are variable, even in successive attacks in the same patient: sometimes the emphasis may be on the scotomatous manifestations, sometimes on the aphasic, sometimes on the affective, and sometimes otherwise, allowing as great a variety of "equivalents" as we have encountered in the decompositions and recompositions of the common migraine. Thus, migraine aura, like common migraine, has a *composite* structure; it is put together from a variety of components or *modules* arranged in innumerable different patterns.

It must also be emphasized that migraine aura has a *sequence* like common migraine, and cannot be adequately portrayed in terms of the symptoms present at any one time. We may readily recognize both excitatory and inhibitory phases, the former manifest as scintillations and paresthesia, diffuse sensory enhancement, arousal of consciousness and muscular tonus, and so on, and the latter as negative hallucinations, loss of muscular tone, syncope, and some others. The time scale of the aura is much contracted, the sequence of excitation-inhibition-reexcitation, and so forth, taking only twenty to thirty minutes, as opposed to a cycle of hours or days in a common migraine. Finally, we observe that the symptoms of the aura are central and cerebral, whereas many (but not all) of the symptoms of a common migraine are peripheral and vegetative.

Incidence of Migraine Aura

The incidence of migraine aura is almost impossible to assess. It has been estimated that the incidence of classical migraine is less than one percent in the general population, but this gives us no information concerning the incidence of isolated auras, which may not form the grounds of complaint, or be recognized for what they are by either patient or physician.* Thus Alvarez, in a study of over 600 migraine scotomata, estimated that more than twelve percent of his male patients experienced solitary scotomata. In a more sophisticated group (comprised of forty-four physicians) he found that no less than 87 percent of them had experienced "many solitary scotomata with never a headache." If we also take into consideration the occurrence of negative scotomata (which may pass unnoticed by the patient), of isolated paresthesia, attacks of faintness and drowsiness, of altered affect, and of disordered highest functions, and other phenomena—all of which may occur as manifestations of aura, but by their subtlety or ambiguity elude diagnosis—we may reasonably suspect the incidence of migraine aura to be far in excess of the quoted incidence of classical migraine.

The Differential Diagnosis of Migraine Aura: Migraine versus Epilepsy

The differentiation of migraine aura from other paroxysmal states, in particular epilepsy, is a vital diagnostic exercise. It is frequently asserted, either on clinical or statistical grounds, that the two maladies are closely related to each other; opposed to this school of opinion are those who vehemently deny the existence, or even the possibility, of such a relation. It is evident that there is much doubt (assertion and denial imply doubt), and that the matter carries too great an emotional charge for cool discussion. Doubt springs from the inadequacy of our definitions, and emotional charge from the sinister and pejorative reputation so often attached to epilepsy. We have already referred to certain clinical associations (Gowers' "borderlands of epilepsy," and Lennox's "hybrid seizures"), and the time has come to clarify the meaning of such terms.

The crux of the matter, as Hughlings Jackson repeatedly stated, lies in the distinction between two frames of reference: roughly speaking, theory and practice. Thus Jackson writes:

*E.g., I happened to be discussing the subject with a colleague, a zoologist, who immediately recognized my diagram of a scintillating scotoma, and said: "I often had it as a young man, usually when I was in bed at night. I was delighted by the colors and their expansion—it reminded me of the opening of a flower. It was never succeeded by a headache or other symptoms. I presumed everybody saw such things—it never occurred to me that it was a 'symptom' of anything."

While scientifically migraine is, I think, to be classified with epilepsies . . . it would be as absurd to classify it along with ordinary cases of epilepsy as to class whales with other mammals for purposes of practical life. A whale is in law a fish; in zoology it is a mammal.

In practice, it is easy to differentiate migraines from epilepsies in the vast majority of cases. Doubt is only likely to arise in the case of complex auras, especially if they occur as isolated events. Doubt may be exacerbated if there is any personal or family history of epilepsy, if the patient loses consciousness during the aura, and, above all, if he is alleged to have had a convulsion while unconscious. It may be instructive, therefore, to compare certain specific phenomena as they occur in epilepsy and in migraine, and in so doing we may reinforce personal experience with the most reliable figures in the older literature—those of Liveing (1873) in relation to migraine, and of Gowers (1881) in relation to epilepsy.

Visual symptoms are far commoner in migraine, and often assume a very specific form—scintillating and negative scotomata—not seen in epileptic auras; visual symptoms were recorded in 62 percent of Liveing's cases (this included both common and classical varieties, but predominantly the latter), but only 17 percent of Gowers' cases. *Paresthesia* of Jacksonian distribution occur with somewhat greater frequency in migraine (35 percent of Liveing's cases, 17 percent of Gowers'), but are very rarely bilateral in epilepsy, whereas they are frequently so in migraine, especially in the lip and tongue areas; a crucial differentiation is given by the rate of passage of such paresthesia, those of migraine being, very roughly, a hundred times slower than their epileptic counterparts. *Convulsions* are common in epilepsy, but are so rare in migraine as to cast doubt on its diagnosis: post-ictal weakness is the rule in motor epilepsies, but does not occur in migraines save in the very special case of hemiplegic attacks (see following chapter). *Loss of consciousness* is common in epilepsy (it occurred in 50 percent of Gowers' 505 cases), but it is a distinct rarity in migraine; further it is generally abrupt in onset in epilepsy (save in psychomotor seizures), but gradual in onset in migraine. Complex *alterations of higher integrative functions and affect* are recorded by both authors as occurring in more than 10 percent of their patients; it is, however, rare for the dreamy or dissociated states of migraine aura to reach the intensity of those

occurring in certain temporal lobe seizures (e.g., automatism followed by amnesia), and, conversely, rare for epileptics to experience
the protracted delirium or quasi-delirium which may accompany
and greatly outlast migraine auras.

By these and similar criteria we may achieve diagnostic certainty,
or at least diagnostic probability, in a majority of cases. There
remain for consideration those patients who appear to experience
both epileptic and migrainous attacks, or the evolution of one into
the other; those patients with true "hybrid" attacks; and, finally,
those patients in whom attacks are of such ambiguous nature as to
defeat clinical diagnostic methods. The reader must be referred to
the exceedingly detailed writings of Gowers (1907) and of Lennox
and Lennox (1960) for a full discussion of this twilight region, and
for a tally of case histories which plays havoc with our rigid
nosologies.

Gowers provides several case histories of migraines and epilepsies
alternating in the same patient, one set of symptoms usually ousting
the other at different periods in the life-history. More dramatic are
his cases "in which there is an actual passage of the symptoms of
one into the other": thus in one such patient, a girl who had been
subject to classical migraines since the age of five, the headache component by degrees disappeared and was replaced by convulsions. (We will recollect that Aretaeus first described such
a hybrid attack of migraine spectrum followed by convulsion.)
Gowers ascribes the onset of epilepsy in such cases to the effects of
migrainous pain and cerebral disturbance: Liveing, more plausibly,
if more enigmatically, speaks of the perpetual possibility of "transformations" from one paroxysm to another.

Lennox and Lennox provide more case histories of this type, in
which the epileptic component, where present, could be further
substantiated by electroencephalographic findings. In one such case
a patient with elaborate visual disturbances (yellow whirling stars
and Lilliputian vision) might suffer either a *grand mal* convulsion
or a classical migraine headache in their wake. Another patient
with protracted visual and paresthetic symptoms would then suffer
severe headache, and, finally, a generalized convulsion, the
headache still being present after the convulsion had terminated.
Lennox terms this attack a "migralepsy."

It is clear that in a majority of instances questioning and observation will resolve the problem as to whether an acute paroxysmal attack is migrainous, epileptic, or of any other type. There are occasions, however, when the greatest clinical acumen may fail to clarify the issue: we have described, for example, migraine auras characterized by hallucinations of smell, feelings of *déjà vu,* and sometimes forced reminiscence and forced affect, which may be indistinguishable from epileptic "uncinate attacks" unless further differential features are present.

The most ambiguous region is that occupied by paroxysmal dreamlike or trancelike states accompanied by intense affect (terror, rapture, etc.) and elaborate alterations of highest mental functions. The differential diagnosis in such cases must include the following states:

> migraine aura
> epileptic aura or psychomotor seizure
> hysterical trances or psychotic states
> toxic, metabolic, or febrile delirious or hysteroid states
> sleep and arousal disorders: for example, nightmares, daymares, atypical narcolepsies or sleep paralyses

We may thus encounter what has already been described in relation to the differential diagnosis of certain migraine equivalents: a region where a number of clinical syndromes appear to coalesce and to become indistinguishable from one another with the means at our disposal. Finally the problem may cease to be one of clinical or physiological differentiation, and become one of semantic decision: we cannot name what we cannot individuate.

Either a thing has properties which no other thing has, and then one has to distinguish it straight away from the others by a description and refer to it; or, on the other hand, *there are several things which have the totality of their properties in common, and then it is not possible to point to any one of them.*

For if a thing is not distinguished by anything, I cannot distinguish it—for otherwise it would be distinguished.

—Wittgenstein

Appendix: The Visions of Hildegard

The religious literature of all ages is replete with descriptions of "visions," in which sublime and ineffable feelings have been accompanied by the experience of radiant luminosity (William James speaks of "photism" in this context). It is impossible to ascertain, in the vast majority of cases, whether the experience represents a hysterical or psychotic ecstasy, the effects of intoxication, or an epileptic or migrainous manifestation. A unique exception is provided in the case of Hildegard of Bingen (1098–1180), a nun and mystic of exceptional intellectual and literary powers, who experienced countless "visions" from earliest childhood to the close of her life, and has left exquisite accounts and figures of these in the two manuscript codices which have come down to us—*Scivias* and *Liber divinorum operum simplicis hominis*.

A careful consideration of these accounts and figures leaves no room for doubt concerning their nature: they were indisputably migrainous, and they illustrate, indeed, many of the varieties of visual aura earlier discussed. Singer (1958), in the course of an extensive essay on Hildegard's visions, selects the following phenomena as most characteristic of them:

In all a prominent feature is a point or a group of points of light, which shimmer and move, usually in a wave-like manner, and are most often interpreted as stars or flaming eyes [*figure 6b*]. In quite a number of cases one light, larger than the rest, exhibits a series of concentric circular figures of wavering form [*figure 6a*]; and often definite fortification figures are described, radiating in some cases from a colored area [*figures 6c and 6d*]. Often the lights gave that impression of *working*, boiling or fermenting, described by so many visionaries. . . .

Hildegard writes:

The visions which I saw I beheld neither in sleep, nor in dreams, not in madness, nor with my carnal eyes, nor with the ears of the flesh, nor in hidden places; but wakeful, alert, and with the eyes of the spirit and the inward ears, I perceived them in open view and according to the will of God.

One such vision, illustrated by a figure of stars falling and being quenched in the ocean (*figure 6b*), signifies for her the "Fall of the Angels":

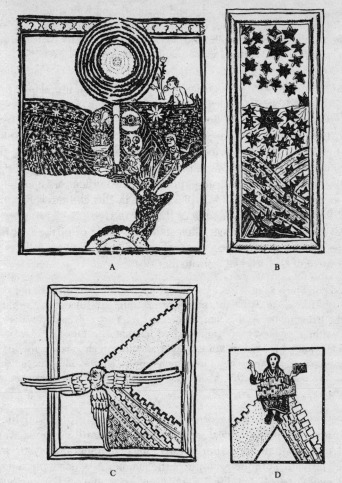

Figure 6. Varieties of migraine hallucination represented in the
visions of Hildegard

Representations of migrainous visions, from a MS of Hildegard's *Scivias*, written at
Bingen about 1180. In *figure 6a*, the background is formed of shimmering stars set
upon wavering concentric lines. In *figure 6b*, a shower of brillant stars (phosphenes)
is extinguished after its passage—the succession of positive and negative scotoma: in
figures 6c and *6d*, Hildegard depicts typically migrainous fortification figures radiating from a central point, which, in the original, is brilliantly luminous and colored
(see text).

I saw a great star most splendid and beautiful, and with it an exceeding multitude of falling stars which with the star followed southwards. . . . And suddenly they were all annihilated, being turned into black coals . . . and cast into the abyss so that I could see them no more.

Such is Hildegard's allegorical interpretation. Our literal interpretation would be that she experienced a shower of phosphenes in transit across the visual field, their passage being succeeded by a negative scotoma. Visions with fortification figures are represented in her *Zelus Dei* (*figure 6c*) and *Sedens Lucidus* (*figure 6d*), the fortifications radiating from a brilliantly luminous and (in the original) shimmering and colored point. These two visions are combined in a composite vision (frontispiece), and in this she interprets the fortifications as the *aedificium* of the city of God.

Great rapturous intensity invests the experience of these auras, especially on the rare occasions when a second scotoma follows in the wake of the original scintillation:

The light which I see is not located, but yet is more brilliant than the sun, nor can I examine its height, length or breadth, and I name it "the cloud of the living light." And as sun, moon, and stars are reflected in water, so the writings, sayings, virtues and works of men shine in it before me. . . .

Sometimes I behold within this light another which I name "the living Light itself." . . . And when I look upon it every sadness and pain vanishes from my memory, so that I am again as simple maid and not as an old woman.

Invested with this sense of ecstasy, burning with profound theophorous and philosophical significance, Hildegard's visions were instrumental in directing her toward a life of holiness and mysticism. They provide a unique example of the manner in which a physiological event, banal, hateful, or meaningless to the vast majority of people, can become, in a privileged consciousness, the substrate of a supreme ecstatic inspiration. One must go to Dostoyevski, who experienced on occasion ecstatic epileptic auras to which he attached momentous significance, to find an adequate historical parallel:

There are moments, and it is only a matter of five or six seconds, when you feel the presence of the eternal harmony . . . a terrible thing is the frightful clearness with which it manifests itself and the rapture with which it fills you. If this state were to last more than five seconds, the soul could not endure it and would have to disappear. During these five seconds I live a whole human existence, and for that I would give my whole life and not think that I was paying too dearly.

Classical Migraine

A lengthy consideration of migraine aura has left us with relatively little to say about classical migraine. A certain proportion of patients may proceed from the aura to a protracted vascular headache, with nausea, abdominal pain, autonomic symptoms, and so forth, of many hours' duration. The repertoire of such symptoms in a classical migraine is no different from that of a common migraine, and requires, therefore, no specific description.

There tend, however, to be some general differences of format. Classical migraines tend to be more compact and intense than common migraines, and rarely have a duration in excess of twelve hours; frequently the attack may last only two or three hours. The termination of the attack may be similarly incisive, and followed by an abrupt return to normal function, or postmigrainous rebound. As Liveing writes in this context:

The abrupt transition from intense suffering to perfect health is very remarkable. A man . . . finds himself, with little or no warning, completely disabled, the victim of intense bodily pain, mental prostration, and perhaps hallucinations of sense or idea . . . and in this state he remains the greater part of the day; and yet towards its close . . . he awakes a different being, in possession of all his faculties, and able to join an evening's entertainment, to get up a brief, or take part in a debate.

The protracted course of some common migraines, in which the patient may spend day after day in a state of wretched malaise, is rarely seen in a classical attack.

We will consider the frequency and antecedents of migraines in Part II, but we may notice, at this point, that classical migraines tend to be less frequent than common migraines, and often have a "paroxysmal" rather than a "reactive" quality. This does not represent an absolute "rule," but is nevertheless a frequent distinguishing characteristic of the two types of attack.

There is a strong tendency for patients to adhere to a given clinical pattern; patients with classical migraine rarely have common migraines, and vice versa. Again, there are no absolutes—I have seen at least thirty patients who suffer from both types of attack, the two types existing either concurrently or in alternation.

We have already noted that some patients who were prone to classical migraines at one time may "lose" the headache component, and thereafter suffer from isolated auras (see case 14).* Conversely, there are also a considerable number of patients who lose their auras, and thereafter suffer from attacks similar to common migraine.

The headache of a classical migraine characteristically comes on as the aura draws to its close, and rapidly attains climactic intensity. It may affect either or both sides of the head, and its location bears no consistent relationship to the lateralization of the aura. Indeed, further attacks of aura may occur after the headache has been established. We have seen that the aura and the headache stages may become spontaneously dissociated in a variety of circumstances (see case 11, for example), and they are also readily separated by ergot derivatives and other drugs which "abort" attacks of classical migraine.

We thus have a number of reasons for thinking classical migraine as a sort of hybrid in which the aura and the headache stages have a contingent link, or tendency to be associated, but no necessary or essential connection.

---

*A number of patients who have suffered from classical migraines for many years have proceeded to "lose" their headaches while under my care, despite the fact that no specific medication has been given. I suspect that this modification of migraine-format is due to suggestion, a consequence of my showing extreme interest in their aura symptoms, and rather less interest in their headaches.

4

Migrainous Neuralgia ("cluster headache")— Hemiplegic Migraine— Ophthalmoplegic Migraine— Pseudomigraine

These variants of migraine are considered in the course of a single chapter because they have one characteristic in common: the occurrence of neurological deficits which may be of considerable duration. Other than this accidental characteristic, they bear no special affinity to one another.

Migrainous Neuralgia

Migrainous neuralgia has been redescribed and renamed a dozen times since Möllendorf's original account in 1867. Among its synonyms are "ciliary neuralgia," "sphenopalatine neuralgia," "Horton's cephalalgia," "histamine headache," and "cluster headache."

The syndrome is a very distinctive one, and its affinities to other forms of migraine have appeared questionable to some observers. There is usually an extremely acute onset of pain referred to the temple and the eye on one side; less frequently, pain may be felt in or behind the ear, or in the cheek and nose. The intensity of the pain may be overwhelming (one patient described it to me as an "orgasm of pain"), and may drive patients into a frenzy. Whereas the majority of migraine patients sit or lie down, or wish to do so, the sufferer from migrainous neuralgia tends to pace up and down in a fury, clutching the affected eye and groaning. I have even seen patients beat their heads against the wall during an attack.

The pain tends to be accompanied (and, on occasion, preceded) by a number of striking local symptoms and signs. The affected eye becomes bloodshot and waters, and there is blockage or catarrh of the nostril on the same side. Sometimes the attack is accompanied or heralded by a flow of thick saliva, rarely by recurrent coughing. There may be a partial or complete *Horner's syndrome* on the affected side, and this may occasionally persist as a permanent neurological residue. The duration of the attacks may be as little as two minutes, and is rarely more than two hours.

A majority of attacks are nocturnal and wake the patient from deep sleep; some come on within a few minutes of waking in the morning, before the fogs of sleep have lifted; diurnal attacks, when they occur, tend to come during periods of rest, exhaustion, or "let-down." They are uncommon when patients are fully aroused and going "full blast." It is rarely possible to identify any *trigger* of the attacks, other than alcohol: during susceptible periods (see page 113) the sensitivity to alcohol is so consistent that it can afford a diagnostic test when the history is equivocal.

I have seen seventy-four cases of migrainous neuralgia in a total of nearly 1,200 migraine patients. This figure probably conveys a disproportionately high incidence, and reflects the fact that the unfortunate sufferers from this symptom are usually forced to seek medical help, and may wander from one physician to another, finally coming to a headache specialist, in order to secure relief from a stubborn and terrible symptom.

Two other peculiarities of incidence may be noted. Migrainous neuralgia is almost ten times commoner in men than in women (the sex-incidence of other forms of migraine is probably equal), and it is rarely familial; only three of seventy-four cases I have seen had a family background of similar attacks, whereas other forms of migraine are commonly familial.

Finally, we must notice the singular format of attacks in many patients, a format which justifies the name of "cluster headache" for this variant of the syndrome. One sees, in such patients, a close-packed grouping of attacks lasting for several weeks (there may be as many as ten attacks daily), and this is followed by a remission lasting months, or even years. Some patients tend to have annual clusters with some regularity (Easter is the usual cluster season) while others may go ten years or more between clusters. During these remissions, patients appear to be entirely immune from attack, and may, in addition, take indefinite quantities of alcohol with impunity. Sometimes the cluster is of abrupt onset, but more commonly it builds up by degrees to a climactic intensity over the course of a few days. Sometimes there is a distinct prodromal period, in which the patient may note a vague burning or discomfort on one side, not amounting to frank pain. Sometimes the imminence of a cluster is announced by the development of alcohol-sensitivity. Some clusters taper off by degrees, although the usual pattern is of sudden, dramatic cessation of the attacks.

There are other sufferers from migrainous neuralgia who never enjoy the blessing of intermittent remission, but have continued attacks, often several a week, for years on end. Attacks are almost invariably confined to one side; I have seen only two patients who have had attacks on alternating sides. A few patients demonstrate tenderness and induration of a superficial temporal artery during a "cluster," or permanently.

The best evidence for the relation of such attacks to common migraine lies in the occurrence of "transitional" attacks which combine features of both (see case 1, below). Their identification with migraine is further fortified by consideration of their physiological substrates (Part III), and their response to medication (Part IV).

Illustrative Case Histories

Case 1

Atypical cluster attacks. The initial attacks are of lancinating severity, very brief duration, and entirely local in their manifestations. As the cluster proceeds, the individual attacks become longer, less intense in severity, and accompanied by abdominal pain, diarrhea and varied autonomic symptoms, that is, indistinguishable from common migraines. There is intense alcohol-sensitivity during, and only during the clusters. Clusters come annually, with considerable regularity, and have only failed to come at the expected time when this patient was pregnant.

Case 2

A 28-year-old man who had suffered incessant attacks of migrainous neuralgia from the age of 18 to 25, but subsequently differentiated a cluster pattern. His younger brother is similarly affected. This patient provides an instructive account of the times and circumstances at which he is liable to an attack, namely in the middle of the night, when "napping" before the television set, when resting after work or a heavy meal, or following an orgasm.

Case 3

A 40-year-old man with migrainous neuralgia who presents a number of unusual features. Lacrimation constitutes an invariable "warning" of an impending attack, and may precede the onset of pain by one or two hours. The majority of attacks are right-sided, but about one in twenty occurs on the left side. The implacable frequency of his attacks has been successfully broken up by the use of monthly injections of histamine. The histamine-reaction is immediately followed by a true attack of migrainous neuralgia, and this, apparently, "defuses" the patient, exempting him from further attacks until his next injection.

Case 5

A 36-year-old woman who suffers from both classical migraines *and* cluster headache. Her attacks of migrainous neuralgia are invariably nocturnal, and are remarkable for the profuse and viscid salivation which accompanies them.

Case 6

A 47-year-old man, paranoid, masochistic, and depressed. He too suffers from two forms of migraine—attacks of migrainous neuralgia nightly, and attacks of common migraine at weekends. He demonstrates a permanently tender and indurated superficial temporal artery on the affected, right side.

Case 7

A 37-year-old man with a twelve-year history of cluster headache. Each cluster is preceded by a prodromal period of about a week, during which there is a diffuse burning feeling in the right temple and tender induration of the superficial temporal artery on this side. He displays a permanent partial Horner's syndrome. Individual attacks are accompanied by intense restlessness, frequency of urination and polyuria.

Case 8

A 55-year-old man who has suffered from annual clusters of migrainous neuralgia since the age of 12, his sole remission being for a period of five years when he was undergoing psychoanalysis.

Hemiplegic Migraine

The term *hemiplegic migraine* is often loosely used to denote ordinary attacks of classical migraine with transient neurological symptoms, as well as attacks in which a true motor hemiplegia of hours' or days' duration is seen. This type of migraine is exceedingly rare. I have seen only the following two cases:

Case 23

A 43-year-old woman who has had classical migraine since the age of 12 (six to ten attacks yearly), and occasional hemiplegic attacks—five in all. Similar hemiplegic attacks had also occurred in her mother and in a maternal aunt. I was enabled to examine her in one attack, at which time she demonstrated a left-sided hemiparesis with impaired cortical sensation and an extensor plantar response. This hemiparesis cleared in three days. She was subsequently admitted for detailed neurological investigation: angiography and contrast-studies failed to visualize any anatomical lesion.

Case 25

A 14-year-old boy who had suffered repeated "bilious attacks" between the ages of 5 and 11, and infrequent classical migraines of great severity since their termination. The majority of his attacks were precipitated by a combination of extravagant exercise and exertion, and tended to come immediately after cross-country races at school.

A number of his attacks were accompanied by a lower facial weakness of many hours' duration, and on one occasion of three days' duration. The father experienced severe attacks of classical migraine without a facioplegic component.

Ophthalmoplegic Migraine

Ophthalmoplegic migraine is also exceedingly rare (Friedman, Harter and Merritt [1961] were able to find only eight cases in a population of 5,000 migraine patients). The majority of patients have usually experienced many common or classical migraines, of which a few attacks have been followed by ophthalmoplegic symptoms. It need hardly be emphasized that this diagnosis should only be made after careful neurological investigation, and the exclusion of possible anatomical abnormalities (aneurysms, angiomas, etc.).

The third cranial nerve is most frequently involved, but the fourth and sixth nerves may also be affected on occasion, leading to total ophthalmoplegia. These neurological deficits usually take several weeks to clear. Involvement in repeated attacks is always unilateral. It has been suggested that the involvement of cranial nerves is due to edema in the intracavernous portion of the internal carotid artery, but there is no supporting evidence for this supposition.

I have seen two cases of ophthalmoplegic migraine in a total of 1,200 migraine patients:

Case 24

This 34-year-old woman has had infrequent common migraines since childhood, and a total of three ophthalmoplegic attacks at widely separated intervals (1943, 1953 and 1966). All of these were preceded by a series of common migraines of increasing severity, and in rapid succession to one another. The culminating attack would be followed, the next day, by the development of an ophthalmoplegia. In her 1966 attack, a series of intense left-sided headaches was followed by the development of third- and fourth-nerve paralyses. The patient experienced complete ptosis for three weeks, and diplopia for a further month. When I examined her, ten weeks after the start of her ophthalmoplegia, she exhibited a dilated pupil on the affected side, but no ptosis or external palsy. Bilateral carotid angiography, performed during the first of her attacks, had been entirely within normal limits.

Case 73

A 9-year-old girl with attacks of classical migraine since the age of 3. One of her attacks, at the age of 5, had been followed by an ophthalmoplegia of many weeks' duration. Two brothers, both parents, and other close relatives were subject to classical migraine, but none had experienced ophthalmoplegic symptoms.

Pseudomigraine

The diagnosis of migraine is usually made on the basis of a clinical history, supported where possible by observation of the patient during an attack. It is usually good sense to perform a few basic investigations (skull x-rays, EEG, etc.), although these may be expected to be within normal limits in the vast majority, say 99 percent, of all cases. Certain clinical features, such as the apparent onset of migraines late in life, are *ipso facto* suspicious of organic pathology, and must be investigated with unusual care. It is particularly important, in cases of classical migraine, to question the patient carefully regarding the usual locations and qualities of the aura. We have already stressed that most migraine patients experience, at one time or another, auras referred to either or both sides of the visual fields or body surface. Invariable unilaterality of the aura is a suspicious symptom, and constitutes grounds for detailed investigation of the patient. The following case history is instructive in this regard:

Case 26

A 57-year-old woman who gave a history of having had "classical migraines" since the age of 16. She would generally experience six or seven attacks a year, and there had been no recent change in this frequency. A careful interrogation revealed certain unusual features in her auras. Both scotomata and paresthesiae were *invariably* confined to the right side of the visual field and body—the patient was emphatic that they had never occurred on the other side. Further, her paresthesiae had on occasion remained unchanged and static for three hours, without showing any Jacksonian march. (It was pointed out, in the last chapter, that a single sweep of scotoma or paresthesia normally takes twenty to forty minutes.) In view of this minor but important divergence from the usual picture, further investigation was undertaken.

Skull x-rays showed a calcified mass in the left posterior hemisphere. Electroencephalography indicated a slow-wave focus, and brain scan, an increased isotope-uptake in this region. Angiography revealed a massive parieto-occipital angioma in the left hemisphere.

Although it is not our intention to enter into the "differential diagnosis" of vascular headaches—a subject very adequately treated in many textbooks—we may emphasize, by means of a case history, that conditions other than cerebral tumors, malformations or aneurysms may occasionally mimic migraines, or be mistaken for them:

Case 48

A 57-year-old woman developed a persistent and severe throbbing headache located in the left temple and eye. Her local physician diagnosed this as an "atypical migraine," although the patient had never previously suffered from headaches, and prescribed ergot drugs and tranquilizers for the patient. Since her symptoms failed to settle under this regimen, he referred her to me for further investigation. On examination, I found a tender and indurated left temporal artery, early papillitis and some diminution of central visual acuity. A sedimentation rate was at once procured, and found to be 110 mm/hour (Westergren), and the presumptive diagnosis of "temporal arteritis" was made. The patient was at once placed on massive doses of prednisone, and the headache remitted within two days. There was, however, some permanent loss of visual acuity.

Permanent Neurological or Vascular Damage from Migraine

Many patients and some physicians entertain considerable apprehension regarding the likelihood of permanent residual damage from migraine, an apprehension fanned by rare but dramatic case reports (which may be reproduced or distorted in the popular press).

Many of these case reports have probably inculpated migraine as a cause for cerebrovascular accidents, while failing to take into account the possibilities of concomitant hypertension, vascular pathology or coincidence. There *are*, however, a number of case reports (the subject has been reviewed both by Dunning [1942] and by Wolff, among others) in which the relation of permanent or fatal damage due to migraine cannot be doubted. Blindness (consequent upon retinal hemorrhage or infarction), hemianopia, hemiplegia and hemisensory deficits, subarachnoid and cerebral hemorrhages have all been recorded in this small but sinister literature.

Nevertheless, it cannot be stated too strongly that such permanent residues are *rare*. My own experience, no less than a perusal of the literature, has assured me of this: I have interrogated and examined more than twelve hundred patients with migraine, and none of them has ever experienced any permanent damage from a migraine. For all its miseries, migraine is an essentially benign and reversible condition, and it is imperative to reassure all patients of this.

Addendum

In my wish to be reassuring, I may have gone too far in the above. Long lasting neurological deficits, though mercifully rare, have been increasingly recognized in recent years, especially as sequelae to so-called basilar artery migraine (Bickerstaff, *Lancet* [1961] 1:15) and "complicated migraine" (G. W. Bruyn, *Handbook of Clinical Neurology*).

5

The Structure of Migraine

We have now surveyed the major patterns of migraine, in all their
bewildering variety and heterogeneity. We must pause, at this
point, to take stock, and to simplify. A clear-cut definition of migraine retreats before us as we advance into the subject, but we are
equipped now to formulate a number of general statements, and to
trace the basic design or *structure* of migraine, as this underlies its
innumerable clinical expressions and permutations.

We have observed that all migraines are composed of many
symptoms (and physiological alterations) proceeding in unison: at
each and every moment the structure of migraine is *composite*.
Thus, a common migraine is fabricated of many components surrounding the cardinal and defining symptom of headache. Migraine
equivalents are composed of essentially similar components aggre-
gated and emphasized in other ways. The structure of migraine aura
is similarly composite. Given the components *a*, *b*, *c* . . . we may
encounter innumerable combinations and permutations of these: *a*
plus *b*, *a* plus *c*, *a* plus *b* plus *c*, *b* plus *c* . . . and so on. It again
needs to be stressed, as at the end of chapter 2, that though the
physiological structure of migraine may be composite, it is experienced by the patient as a unity or whole, with a unitary character
or physiognomy of its own. We may analyze a migraine into parts;
the *patient* experiences it as a seamless whole.

Beneath these variable and disjunctive components, we may recognize the occurrence of other, relatively stable features, occurring
in constant conjunction: these constitute, as it were, the *core* of
the migraine structure. It is in the middle range—between the

vegetative disturbances and the cortical disturbances—that the *essential* features of migraine may be found: alterations of conscious level, of muscular tonus, of sensory vigilance, and the like. We may subsume these under a single term: they represent disorders of *arousal*. In extremely severe attacks, the degree of arousal occurring in the earlier or prodromal stages of the migraine may proceed to agitation or even frenzy, while the ensuing stages may be marked by a subsidence into lethargy or even stupor. In milder attacks the disorders of arousal may be overshadowed by the presence of pain or other florid symptoms, and thus be overlooked by patient and physician. Disorders of arousal, mild or severe, appear to be invariable features of all migraines.

Each stage in the course of a migraine is marked by the concurrence of symptoms at *different functional levels*, in particular the concurrence of physical and of emotional symptoms. These cannot be described in terms of one another: each level must be described by a language appropriate to it. Thus migraine is conspicuously a psychophysiological event, and requires for its understanding a sort of mental diplopia (to adopt Jackson's term) and a double language. The most primitive symptoms of migraine are both physical *and* emotional: thus *nausea*, for example, is both a sensation and a "state of mind" (the literal and figurative uses of the word nausea are of equal antiquity); nausea is in the region where the separateness of sensations and emotions has not yet been established. More complex symptoms have become dichotomized, so to speak, so that we may recognize, at every stage throughout an attack, a constant concomitance and paralleling of physical and emotional symptoms. We may, for example, portray the sequence of a typical (prototype) migraine in terms of the following five stages:

(1) The initial *excitement* or excitation of an attack (provided either externally by a provocative stimulus, or internally by an aura), in which the emotional aspects may be experienced as rage, elation, or other events, and the physiological aspects as heightened sensory perception, scintillating scotomata, paresthesiae, and other experiences.

(2) A state of *engorgement* (sometimes termed the prodrome, sometimes simply the earlier stages of an attack), characterized by the occurrence of visceral distension and stasis, vascular dilatation, fecal retention, fluid retention, muscular tension, and so on, and,

concurrently with these symptoms, feelings of emotional tension, anxiety, restlessness, irritability, and the like.

(3) A state of *prostration* (frequently isolated by medical observation, and termed the "attack proper"), in which the affective experience is one of apathy, depression, and retreat, while its physical concomitants are experienced as nausea, malaise, drowsiness, faintness, muscular slackness and weakness, and similar troubles.

(4) The state of recovery or *resolution*, which may be achieved abruptly (crisis) or gradually (lysis). In the case of the former, there may occur a violent visceral ejaculation, such as vomiting or sneezing, or a sudden excess of emotion, or both together; in the case of the latter, a variety of secretory activities (diuresis, diaphoresis, involuntary weeping, etc.) are accompanied by a concurrent melting away, or catharsis, of the existing emotional symptoms.

(5) A stage of *rebound* (if the attack has been brief and compact), in which feelings of euphoria and renewed energy are accompanied by great physical well-being, increased muscular tonus and alertness: generalized arousal.

This remarkable synchronization of affect and somatic symptoms allows us to define the psychophysiological state of a migraine, at any given time, in terms of mood and of autonomic status (or, more accurately, arousal or nervous "tuning": concepts considered fully in Part III). Thus we can conveniently depict the typical course of a migraine on a "map" in which affect and arousal have been selected as coordinates (*figure 7*).

We may comment very briefly on the type of relation which may exist between these somatic and emotional symptoms of a migraine, while deferring full consideration of this topic until much later (Part III). When considering the problem of fluid retention in migraine attacks, we noted Wolff's conclusions, based on painstaking experiment, that fluid retention and vascular headache were concomitant but not causally related to each other; the same is largely true of concomitant emotional and somatic symptoms. Their concurrence, if it cannot be explained in terms of direct causality (the physical symptoms causing the emotional symptoms, or vice versa), must either be traced to a common antecedent cause, or to a symbolic linkage. No other possibilities exist.

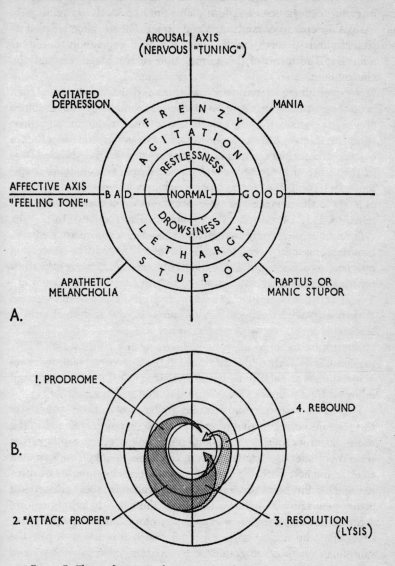

Figure 7. The configuration of migraine, in relation to mood and arousal

We must return now to the general problem of categorizing the migraine experience, and formulating more exactly its relation to idiopathic epilepsy, fainting, vagal attacks, acute affective disturbances, and so forth, with which we have repeatedly noted its affinities. The terms of this formulation, at this stage, can only be clinical ones.

We recognize a migraine as being constituted by certain symptoms of a certain duration in a certain sequence. The structure of a migraine is extremely variable, but it is variable in only three ways. First, the entire course of the attack is variable in *length*: the overall structure of a migraine may be condensed or extended (it is in this sense that Gowers speaks of vagal attacks as extended epilepsies); second, the course of an attack may be enacted at a variety of *levels* in the nervous system—from the level of cortical hallucinations to that of peripheral autonomic disturbances; third, the symptoms at each level may present themselves in many different *combinations and permutations*. Therefore, instead of conceiving migraine as a very specific and stereotyped event, we must rather envisage a broad *region* encompassing the entire repertoire of migraine and migraine-like attacks; within this region, the migraine structure may be modulated in duration, in "vertical level" and in "collateral level," to use Jackson's terms.

The sequence of a full-fledged migraine (i.e., one which is not prematurely terminated, and of which the inaugural stages are recognized) has essentially two stages: a stage of excitation or arousal, followed by a protracted stage of inhibition or "derousal."

It is in these terms that we may first perceive the proximity of the migraine cycle to that of epilepsy, on the one hand, and to the more leisurely cycles of waking and sleep, on the other; the prominent affective components of migraines demand comparison, more remotely, with the excitatory and inhibitory phases of some psychoses. We have observed the occurrence of many transitional states between all of these: the occurrence of "migralepsies," insomniac and hypomanic states preceding migraines and epilepsies, dreamlike and nightmarish auras, apathetic depression during the inhibitory stage of migraine, the occurrence of somnolent and stuporous migraines, the inauguration of migraines during sleep, their abortion by brief sleep, and, finally, the long sleep which characteristically follows severe migraines and epilepsies. In all cases we may see the inhibitory states as morbid variations or caricatures of normal sleep, following upon inordinate excitations (migrainous prodromes and excitements, epileptic convulsions, psychotic agitations), as normal sleep succeeds the activities of the waking day. Gowers placed migraines, faints, sleep disorders, and like occurrences in the "borderland" of epilepsy; we can with equal justice reverse his words, and locate migraine and migrainelike reactions in the borderland of sleep.

It is important to observe that migraine is no more a suspension of all physical and mental activities than sleeping, or psychotic stupors; it is charged, on the contrary, with activities of an inward, private kind. Inhibition at one level releases excitations at other levels. The diminution of motor activity and external ties during a migraine is matched by a great increase in internal activities, vegetative symptoms and their attendant, regressive affects—a paradoxical combination of inner violence and outer detachment—analogous to the dreaming of paradoxical sleep, or the concealed agitations and hallucinations of psychotic stupors.

Gowers, observing the gradual or sudden transformations of one type of migraine into another, or of migraines into epilepsies, fainting attacks, and so forth, concluded: "We can perceive the mysterious relation, but we cannot explain it." We can do no more, at this stage, than point out that all such attacks share a certain formal resemblance in structure, merging into one another, and into the region of migraine. We cannot explore the "mysterious relation" any further without considering the *functions* of migraine and of other paroxysmal reactions which may take its place. We must move ahead, therefore, and learn when and why migraines occur.

Part II

The OCCURRENCE
of MIGRAINE

Introduction

Many patients consider their migraines to occur "spontaneously" and without cause. Such a view leads, scientifically, to absurdity, emotionally, to fatalism, and therapeutically, to impotence. We must assume that all attacks of migraine have real and discoverable determinants, however difficult their elucidation may be.

The determinants of migraine are almost infinite in number, and may present themselves in many different combinations. We may simplify their discussion, as Willis did three centuries ago, by distinguishing predisposing, exciting and accessory causes of migraine. Thus among these Willis recognized the following determinants:

An evil or weak constitution of the parts . . . sometimes innate and hereditary . . . an irritation in some distant member or viscera . . . changes of season, atmospheric states, the great aspects of the sun and moon, violent passions, and errors in diet . . .

We can never predict the occurrence of a migraine with certainty, but our inability to do so reflects only the limitations of our knowledge. It may indeed be certain that if conditions $a, b, c, d, \ldots$ and on and on, are fulfilled, that a migraine will inevitably follow, but we are rarely if ever in possession of *all* the relevant knowledge. Thus we are reduced to speaking in terms of propensities and probabilities.

6

The Predisposition to Migraine

We are accustomed to think of any particular response as either learned or innate, which is apt to be a source of confusion in thinking about such things. . . . Is the response inherited, or acquired? The answer is, Neither: either Yes or No would be very misleading.

—Hebb

If we say of X that he is an epileptic, we make two assertions, that he has seizures, and that he has a propensity towards seizures. The latter is considered to be inherent within him; we may label this inherent propensity an epileptic predisposition, or constitution. It may further be considered that his predisposition is not only inherent, but immutable ("once an epileptic, always an epileptic"), and as such condemn him to a lifetime of caution, anticonvulsants, driving restrictions, and so on. A correlate of these assumptions may be the identification of pathognomonic "signs" of an epileptic constitution—epileptic stigmata.

These propositions are of great historical antiquity, and receive only partial support from admissible data; such truth as they do contain is clearly inflated by emotional bias. Similar assertions are frequently made with regard to "schizophrenic predisposition," and these too must be, and have been, subjected to the most critical scrutiny. These two examples may serve to introduce the subject of migraine predisposition which, if it lacks the pejorative undertones of the commonly held opinions on epileptic or schizophrenic predisposition, will reveal itself as even more complex in its implications.

130

The notion of migraine predisposition rests on three groups of data: first and foremost, studies on the familial incidence of migraine, and subsidiary to this, studies designed to expose pathognomonic signs of the predisposition, and to discover substrative "factors" or "traits" in migrainous and premigrainous populations. The basic assumption, of course, is that migraine is a clearly defined "disease" analogous, for example, to sickle-cell disease which will occur in persons with sickle-cell trait, and only in such persons, when certain other conditions are fulfilled.

The Overall Incidence of Migraine

Headache is the commonest complaint which patients bring to physicians, and migraine is the commonest functional disorder by which patients are afflicted. Figures are only available on the incidence of migraine headache (cephalgic migraine), and these vary between estimates of 5 percent and 20 percent for its incidence in the general population. Balyeat (1933) found an incidence of 9.3 percent in a population of almost 3,000 persons whom he interrogated. Lennox and Lennox (1960) found that migraine headache occurred in 6.3 percent of medical students, nurses and non-epileptic patients whom they questioned. Fitz-Hugh's (1940) figure is as high as 22 percent. Many further figures are cited and discussed in Wolff's monograph.

A general observation must be made concerning all such incidence figures. The terms of interrogation exclude many categories of patient and of migraine, for example, those whose attacks are infrequent and unremembered, those whose attacks are mild and undiagnosed, and, not least, the many patients who experience attacks of migraine equivalent or isolated auras, and for this reason are not considered in the same frame of reference. We may assert that a substantial minority, perhaps one-tenth of the population, experience fairly common and readily recognized cephalgic migraines. We may suspect that many more experience occasional or mild migraines, migraine equivalents, or migraine auras. Certain forms of migraine, it would seem, are much rarer. It has been stated that the incidence of classical migraine is not above 1 percent in the general population (probably an underestimate); migrainous neuralgia is rarer still, and the hemiplegic and ophthalmoplegic forms of migraine are excessively rare, and are unlikely to be seen in a lifetime of practice by the average general physician.

Familial Occurrence and Inheritance of Migraine

It has long been held, and with good reason, that migraine has a strong tendency to run in certain families, and there are innumerable clinical and statistical studies which substantiate this fact. Lennox (1941), reviewing a massive population of patients with migraine (headache), noted that 61 percent of them described a parent as having been affected with migraine, whereas only 11 percent of a control group reported close familial involvement. Friedman has estimated that 65 percent of migraine sufferers seen in a headache clinic give a family history of migraine. The *fact* of frequent familial incidence is indisputable; the interpretation of this fact is far from clear.

The most ambitious and the most sophisticated of these comparative statistical studies is that of Goodell, Lewontin, and Wolff (1954). These workers selected for study 119 patients with "severe headaches recurring usually over many years," and submitted all of these to close interrogation with regard to the incidence of migraine headaches in other members of their families (no distinction was made, for the purpose of this inquiry, between classical and common migraine). It was found, in a comparison of the offspring in these migrainous families, that 28.6 percent of those with neither parent affected had migraine, 44.2 percent of those with one migrainous parent had migraine, and 69.2 percent of those with both parents affected had migraine. Goodell and others, comparing the observed with the expected incidence in the 832 offspring considered, concluded that "there is less than one chance in a thousand that such deviations [from the expected incidence] would occur if the assumption of no inheritance were true . . . Furthermore, it is reasonable to assume that migraine is due to a recessive gene whose penetrance is approximately 70 percent."

We must regard this conclusion as highly suspect and even absurd, despite the thoroughness and elegance of the study. There are at least three hidden assumptions of considerable dubiety, the first relating to sampling, the second to the homogeneity of the population studied, and the third, the most important, to the necessarily ambiguous interpretation of any study of this type. First, only patients with severe, recurrent, long-standing migraine headache were studied, and interrogation concerning affected relatives was similarly framed in terms of these criteria. It is clear, therefore, that if mild or unremembered or infrequent attacks of migraine headache had occurred, or if migraine equivalent or migraine aura had instead been present, the figures of incidence might be very different from the ones obtained. Second, it is assumed, wholly without justification, that the population considered was genetically homogeneous with regard to migraine, that is, that all migraines considered, whether of classical, common, or any other type, were genetically equivalent for purposes of the study. Third, and most crucially, *familial incidence does not necessarily imply inheritance.* A family is not only a source of genes but an environmental circumstance of enormous potency.* Goodell and others are not unaware of this reservation but they do not take it seriously. It must, however, be taken extremely seriously in view of the evidence (to be discussed in later chapters) that migraine reactions are readily adopted, learned, and emulated within the family environment. A rigorous genetic study would have to concern itself with offspring of migrainous parents reared by nonmigrainous foster-parents or, ideally, with the incidence of migraine in identical twins separated at birth. No method less stringent is adequate to distinguish the effects of "nature" versus "nurture" in a reaction as complex and multiply determined as migraine. Without such controls, statistical studies of migraine (as of schizophrenia) cannot claim to do more than quantify what one already knows, that migraine tends to be commoner in certain families. They *cannot* establish any genetic basis, let alone so elementary (and inherently improbable) a basis as a single gene with partial penetrance.

If the ambiguities of sampling and symptom-variability are reduced, and if particularly rare forms of migraine are studied, the likelihood of a hereditary basis may be more plausibly stated. Thus

---

*An instructive example of "pseudoheredity" in the determination of complex psychophysiological reactions is Friedman's finding that not only 65 percent of migraine patients, but 40 percent of patients with tension-headaches, give a family history of their respective symptoms. It has never been suggested (nor is it likely to be suggested) that tension headaches have a genetic basis, but clearly they are adopted in households where this is the family "style."

classical migraine is, roughly, ten times rarer than common migraine, yet tends to show a more dramatic familial occurrence. Hemiplegic migraine, which can hardly be overlooked or forgotten, tends to remain "true to type," is exceedingly rare in the general population, and is almost always found in the context of heavy familial involvement (Whitty, 1953). I myself have seen a patient with hemiplegic migraine who has four siblings, a parent, an uncle, and a first cousin similarly affected.

The matter is of more than academic importance, for if a patient regards himself as "doomed" to a lifetime of migraine in view of a sinister family background of the disorder, and his physician takes an equally fatalistic view of the matter, the chances of any therapeutic intervention are much reduced. Lennox and Lennox, usually most reasonable, write, "Persons with migraine should think twice before marrying one whose own or whose family history is positive for this disorder." This statement, in view of the degree of doubt concerning genetic factors, and the overwhelming importance of environmental factors, is little short of monstrous.

Signs of the Migrainous Constitution

We understand by the term *sign*, in this context, a clinical characteristic which is highly correlated with the tendency to migraine, and which therefore occurs wih exceptional frequency in most migraine patients and many of their relatives. Some such signs will be regarded as an integral part of the migraine constitution, and other signs may have a fortuitous but exceptionally common linkage with the tendency to migraine. The concealed assumption, in all cases, is that there is a unitary genetic basis—Wolff speaks of a "stock factor"— underlying migraine. Thus, to cite a particularly fantastic example of an alleged migrainous trait:

Further evidence of the stock factor in migraine [writes Wolff] is reported by Erik Ask-Upmark, who made the interesting observation that out of thirty-six patients subject to migraine headache attacks, nine had inverted nipples, as compared with sixty-five persons who were not subject to migraine, in whom there was only one instance of inverted nipples.

The majority of such observations, or theories, envisage a constitutional type with particular physical and emotional characteristics as especially or uniquely prone to migraine. Thus Tourraine and Draper (1943) speak of a "characteristic constitutional type" in which the skull shows acromegaloid traits, the intelligence is outstanding, but the emotional make-up is retarded. Alvarez (1959) discerns as prime characteristics of migrainous women:

a small trim body with firm breasts. Usually these women dress well and move quickly. 95 percent had a quick eager mind and much social attractiveness. . . . Some 28 percent were red-headed, and many had luxuriant hair. . . . These women age well.

Greppi (1955) claims to perceive a migraine "ground," a particular psychophysiological constellation very common among, and peculiar to, sufferers from migraine:

There is a certain delicacy or grace . . . there are signs which indicate the development of an early intelligence and sensibility, of a critical and self-controlled temperament.

These accounts exemplify the "romantic" view of migrainous constitution. It is of more than historical interest that so many authors, from antiquity to the present day, are concerned to present so flattering a picture of the migraineur. Perhaps one may connect this tendency with the fact that most writers on migraine suffer from migraine. At all events, such descriptions are greatly at odds with the traditional accounts of epileptics and the epileptic constitution, with their menacing undertones of hereditary "taint" and constitutional "stigmata."

It is frequently stated that migraines are peculiar to a specific "migraine personality," which is usually portrayed as obsessive, rigid, driving, perfectionistic, and so forth. The adequacy of this concept may be measured by the clinical finding of exceedingly varied emotional backgrounds in migraine patients (see chapter 9), and will receive critical discussion at a later stage (Part III).

Some authors have stated that migraine patients may be placed in one or other of the four traditional psychophysiological categories (either Hippocratic or Pavlovian terms may be employed), a supposition which acquaintance with a handful of migraine patients should dispel. There is, however, some evidence that different styles of migraine may be commoner in particular constitutional types, as du Bois Reymond realized a century ago. Thus patients prone to "red" migraines tend to be overtly excitable and to flush with anger (they are, in Pavlov's terms, "strong excitable types," or "sympathotonic"), while other patients prone to "white" migraines tend to pallor, fainting, and withdrawal reactions in the face of emotional stimuli (being "weak inhibitory types" or "vagotonic"). But no general statement on the subject is applicable to migraine patients in their entirety.

Other workers have suggested that the tendency to migraine may be indicated by a variety of physiological parameters: a particular sensibility to passive motion, heat, exhaustion, and depressant drugs (e.g., alcohol and reserpine); exaggerated cardiovascular reflexes (e.g., pathological carotid sinus sensitivity); anatomical or functional "microcirculatory disorder"; the prevalence of slow-wave cerebral dysrhythmias; and a variety of metabolic and chemical dysfunctions. We can do no more, at the present stage, than state that none of these factors have been shown to be of critical relevance to migraine patients as an overall group, although certain of them may show consistent variations in particular subgroups of migraine sufferers.

Migraine Diathesis and Other Disorders

The notion that there may exist, and the search for, other disorders correlated and connected with migraine diathesis, or predisposition is no more than a logical extension of the considerations already raised, but there are a variety of specific issues which demand separate consideration. The area is one of doubt and dispute.

Before embarking on any general discussion, we must inquire more minutely into the evidence which is available concerning the correlation of migraine with specific disorders. There is general agreement that a history of motion sickness, cyclic vomiting, or bilious attacks, in the earlier years of life is exceptionally common among migraine sufferers, although such tendencies and attacks are "replaced" by the adult migraines, for the most part rather rarely continuing their original intensity throughout life. Provided any statement correlating motion-sickness and migraine is a purely statistical one based on a large population, it cannot be gainsaid. If, however, one departs from a statistical approach and concerns oneself only with individual case histories, it is at once obvious that many patients with migraine (especially those with classical migraine) never experienced motion-sickness or visceral eruptions in their earlier years, and may, indeed, have been exceptionally resistant even to stimuli which produce nausea in a majority of the population; conversely, it is obvious that many children who suffer (enjoy?) cyclic vomiting, motion-sickness, and bilious attacks never develop "adult" migraines later in their lives.

The facts—or, rather, the quoted figures, with their attendant sources of error—are less clear concerning the correlation of migraine with hypertension, allergies, epilepsy, and the like, and we will do no more than cite a handful of investigations from the many hundreds which burden the literature. Gardner, Mountain and Hines (1940) found migraine five times more frequent in a hypertensive population than in a control group without hypertension. These authors display a proper reserve in interpreting their data, accepting as equally admissible the hypothesis of a common genetic factor and that of other shared factors (e.g., the prevalence of chronic inhibited rage among hypertensives and migraineurs). Balyeat (1933) was so struck with the incidence of allergic reactions in migraine patients and their families that he took correlation for identity and claimed that migraine *was* allergic in nature in many cases, a view which has since commanded an astonishing following, despite the fact that Wolff, and others, have shown in critical experiments that migraine is almost never allergic in origin. Lennox and Lennox (1960) have long been concerned with the taboo topic of constitutional relationships between migraine and epilepsy. They find (from a study of over 2,000 epileptics) that 23.9 percent of these have a family history of migraine, a figure substantially in excess of such family histories secured from their control group. They conclude that migraine and epilepsy have not only a common "constitutional" basis, but a related genetic basis.

Migraine in Relation to Age

Constitutional disorders usually manifest themselves relatively early in life. We must inquire whether this is true of migraine. Critchley (1933), in an early paper on the subject, stated: "A person is either afflicted with migrainous diathesis from an early age, or he is completely spared. He is unlikely to acquire the malady in adulthood, . . . " There are many figures in literature which would seem to contradict this supposition. Lennox and Lennox (1960), studying 300 patients with migraine, noted that 37.9 percent had their inaugural attack in the third decade or later.

My own experience (with 1,200 migraine patients, the majority adult) has provided abundant confirmation of the frequency of late-onset migraines, and has further indicated the necessity of breaking down the overall group into smaller, clinically homogeneous subgroups before any meaningful statement can be made. *Classical migraine* has perhaps the greatest propensity to present in youth or early adult life, but I have seen a dozen cases in which an initial attack occurred after the age of 40; the distinctiveness and severity of classical migraines are such that prior attacks would be unlikely to escape the memory. Onset in the middle years is far more frequent in the case of *common migraines*, and of these I have seen at least sixty cases presenting after the age of 40, and perhaps a fifth of these presenting after the age of 50; this clinical pattern is particularly seen in women who may become the victims of migraine during or after menopause. *Migrainous neuralgia*, above all, is notorious for its capacity to come on in later life; I have had one patient who experienced an initial "cluster" at the age of 63, and cases of onset in the mid-seventies have been recorded in the literature. There is indisputably a general tendency for migraine to present early in life and dwindle in frequency in the later years, but this is a rule with frequent and important exceptions.

The concept of migraine diathesis carries the implication that migraine is, in some fashion, latent within the individual, until it is provoked to manifest itself. The following case history illustrates how migraine may remain dormant for the greater part of a lifetime, only springing into action, so to speak, given an extraordinary environmental provocation:

Case 15

This patient, a 75-year-old woman, presented herself with the complaint of severe and frequent classical migraines. She had been experiencing two to three attacks a week, each preceded by unmistakable fortification figures and paresthesiae. Her attacks had come on immediately following the tragic death of her husband in a car accident. She admitted to being intensely depressed and to entertaining suicidal thoughts. I asked her whether she had ever had similar attacks before, and she replied that she had had similar attacks in childhood, but had not experienced one of these, to knowledge, for fifty-two *years* prior to her current paroxysm. Over course of some weeks the patient's depression lifted, with the combined influences of time, psychotherapy, and antidepressant drugs. She "became herself" once more, and her classical migraines disappeared into the limbo where they had been dormant for half a century.

In general, one would be somewhat concerned if auralike symptoms—fortifications, scotomata, phosphenes, and others—were to make their appearance *for the first time* in later life, and one would have to wonder about insufficiencies in the cerebral circulation. In this patient, of course, this was not the situation; indeed, her recollection of identical symptoms fifty years previously put an altogether more benign complexion on the matter, suggesting, as it did, the *return* of something she had had all her life, rather than the development of some new and possibly serious pathology.

A further case history emphasizes, even more forcefully, that a migraine diathesis (granting its reality) may remain latent and unsuspected until late in life:

Case 38

This patient was a 62-year-old woman who had suffered from headaches of overwhelming severity for four months. The first, indeed, was so alarming that her husband, a physician, at once procured her admission to hospital. The suspicion of a subarachnoid hemorrhage or intracranial lesion was entertained, but all investigations were negative, and after three days the attack subsided. A month later she suffered a similar attack, and a month after this a third attack. At this stage I saw her in consultation. I questioned the patient, a very intelligent and reliable witness, and she professed herself certain that she had never experienced any symptoms resembling her current periodic attacks. Struck by their monthly occurrence, I inquired whether she had been placed on any drugs recently, and she at once mentioned that her gynecologist had placed her on a hormone preparation, four months before, to be taken cyclically (the drug was a contraceptive estrogen-progestogen preparation prescribed for postmenopausal symptoms). A comparison of dates revealed that each attack had occurred in the week intervening between the cycles of hormone administration. I advised her to try the effect of omitting the hormone. She did so, and experienced no further attacks.

This matter of *latent* symptoms, tendencies, phenomena, being brought out and made manifest by special circumstances, was something I was able to study carefully in another group of patients—who had had the sleeping-sickness in early life, but could only be given an "awakening" drug half a century later. In *Awakenings*, I described the calling-forth or calling-back by the power of L-Dopa, of long-past physiological disturbances, tics, and specific moods and memories, which had lain dormant in the nervous system for fifty years or more.

General Discussion and Conclusions

This chapter, necessarily has been one of statement and counterstatement, of doubts, hesitations and qualifications. We must now, in conclusion, consider the reasons for doubt which apply to statistical studies on migraine predisposition, and the legitimate meanings which can still be given to this concept.

Our first comments must bear on the *validity of sampling*. If statements concerning the frequency of this or that trait in a population are to be of any value or interest, the population must be a relatively homogeneous one. Such statements with reference to migraine are based on the assumption that migraine is a single disorder with a unitary basis. They present to us a variant of that fiction—the average man: the average migraineur is shown as a hypertensive perfectionist with one inverted nipple, multiple allergies, a background of motion-sickness, two-fifths of a peptic ulcer, and a first cousin with epilepsy. Actual clinical experience soon persuades anyone who works with migrainous patients that they are an exceedingly heterogeneous group. Some have classical migraines, some common: some have striking family histories, many have no family histories, some have allergies, some do not; some react to particular drugs, some do not; some are sensitive to alcohol or passive motion, some are not; some outgrow their attacks at a youthful age, others start them at a later age; some have red migraines and some white; some have prominent visceral components, and others chiefly cephalgic components; some are hyperactive, some are lethargic; some are obsessional, others are sloppy; some are brilliant, and some are simpletons. . . . In short, migraine patients are as remarkable for their diversity as any other section of the population. Such heterogeneity of the population and the symptoms under survey may invalidate and render meaningless any statistical survey, and demand, for investigative purposes, that the clinical material be broken down into smaller and more homogeneous groups. If the data are disparate, they must not be put together for purposes of comparison. We cannot reconcile Critchley's clinical impression of negative correlation between migraine and other disorders with the positive correlations claimed by Graham, Wolff, and others. What we must do is to question the value of any and all such general statements. It is clear to the observant physician (and Critchley has fully concealed this in his many clinical publications) that *some* migraine patients remain strikingly faithful to their migraines, apparently finding in these an adequate outlet and expression of whatever nervous instability or stress is driving them; other patients exhibit protean and sudden transformations from one migraine equivalent to another, or from migraine to asthma, faints, and so forth; and a third group seem to have a wide-open psychosomatic cavity, and embrace any and every functional disorder they can. In some, the image of functional disease is fixed and held from an early stage of life, moored to something unchanging in physical reactivity or emotional demand; in others, continually modulated emotional stresses may play upon a xylophonic reactivity an endless series of illness variations.

Our second concern must be with the *validity of interpretation* of statistical correlations. Let us assume that a particular study has skirted sampling errors and emerged with a correlation coefficient, a figure denoting the coincidence of two factors, *a* and *b*. It may be inferred that *a* causes *b*, that *b* causes *a*, or that both share a common cause. All such inferences, particularly the last, are to be found in the literature on migraine predisposition: thus Balyeat sees allergy as causing migraine, some authors see migraine as causing or favoring cerebrovascular accidents, and a majority of workers hold to the hypothesis of a shared diathesis—Wolff's "stock factor"—which can express itself as migraine or as many other disorders. None of these inferences can be justified on statistical grounds alone. A correlation is no more than a figure of coincidence, and in itself implies no logical connection between the phenomena studied. If a particular group of patients show high incidence of both migraine and hypertension, there may be a dozen reasons for this, and the reasons for their hypertension have no necessary connection with the reasons for their migraine. The high incidence of allergic reactions in migraine patients is very generally conceded, but Balyeat's theory of an allergic causation of migraines is demonstrably in error. We have, in such a case, to fall back upon considerations of biological strategy and analogy, and simply say that allergic and migrainous reactions may serve similar purposes in the organism and thus alternate or coexist as equivalent physiological options.

Our final concern is with the *validity of terms* which have been employed in this area: predisposition, diathesis, constitutional susceptibilities, stock factors, and others. We may accept, with some reservations, that a relatively specific predisposition may exist and be transmitted in cases of hemiplegic migraine and in many, though far from all, cases of classical migraine; but these entities are rare, and constitute less than one-tenth of the overall migraine population. We must express the strongest doubts as to whether there exists any specific predisposition to common migraine, let alone a universal "migraine diathesis." How then shall we explain the apparent limitation of migraine to a section of the population, and its emphasis in certain families?

We can accept no terms except the most vague and general ones at the present time. It seems clear that many migraine patients are distinguished by *something* which is present in greater degree than normal.

The repertoire of this something is very wide. Critchley said that it may manifest itself, in the earlier years, as infantile eczema, motion-sickness, and recurrent spells of vomiting. And to this short list we must add all the varieties of migraine which were considered in Part I of this book, and beyond these the many other paroxysmal reactions—faints, vagal attacks, and the like—with which migraines may coalesce or alternate. It is in these terms—of a multiply determined reaction, with innumerable variations of form and apparently endless plasticity—that the concept of migrainous diathesis must be used, if it is to retain any meaning at all. Moreover, this something permits an infinite number of gradations so that the migraine population, far from being clearly defined and set apart, merges into the general population at every point. Everyone, every organism, must be considered to have the potential for reactions *qualitatively* akin to migraine (see Part III), but this potential is exalted, as it

were, and made specific in a particular fraction of the population.*
The facile assumption of a "migraine diathesis" as something simple,
specific, unitary, quantifiable, or reducible to elementary genetics
explains nothing, answers nothing, and begs every question; worse
still, it obscures the elucidation of the true determining factors of
migraine—in the individual and in his environment—by the use of
a contentless phrase. Certainly there is something in a migraine
patient which makes him more liable to his attacks, but the definition of this something, this predisposition, will demand our exploration of a much wider field of reference than the genetic and statistical
considerations which have been considered in this chapter.

If we hope to understand or treat a patient with migraine, we are
likely to find the circumstances of his life history to be of the greatest
importance in having determined and shaped his symptoms; when
we have exhaustively explored and weighed such environmental
factors, we may legitimately speculate upon the possibilities of
constitutional or hereditary factors. Painstaking exploration of clinical histories is indispensable if we are to avoid the temptations of
purely theoretical concepts—migraine "diathesis," migraine "stock
factor," single-gene inheritance, and so on—which may be no more
than fictions. We must adapt the words with which Freud closed a
famous case history:

I am aware that expression has been given in many quarters to thoughts
. . . which emphasize the hereditary, phylogenetically acquired factor. . . .
I am of the opinion that people have been far too ready to find room for
them and ascribe importance to them. . . . I consider that they are only
admissible when one strictly observes the correct order of precedence, and,
after forcing one's way through the strata of what has been acquired by the
individual, comes at last upon traces of what has been inherited.

*"At one end of the series stand those extreme cases of whom one can say: These
people would have fallen ill whatever happened, whatever they experienced. . . .
At the other end stand cases which call forth the opposite verdict—they would
undoubtedly have escaped illness if life had not put such and such burdens on them.
In the intermediate cases in the series, more or less of the disposing factor . . . is
combined with more or less of the injurious impositions of life" (Freud, *A General
Introduction to Psychoanalysis*, 1920, p. 356).

7

Periodic and
Paroxysmal Migraines

Migraine and Other Biological Cycles

Equilibrium in biological systems is achieved only by the continuous balancing of opposite forces. Frequently it is maintained homeostatically, by continuous small adjustments to a dynamic system. At other times, its achievement depends on profound alterations of the system occurring at intervals, cyclically or sporadically. Some of these cycles are universal, like the alternation of sleeping and waking, while others are manifest in only a fraction of the population, as with cycles of epilepsy, psychosis, and migraine. In all of these cases, the tendency to cycling is inherent in the nervous system, although the innate periodicity may be accessible to a variety of external influences. We will speak, therefore, of "periodic migraine" in considering attacks which occur at fairly regular intervals, *irrespective of the mode of life*, and of "paroxysmal migraines" in regard to apparently spontaneous attacks which occur at irregular or widely separated intervals.

Periodicity, in this sense, may mark the pattern of any form of migraine, but is peculiarly characteristic of classical migraines and of cluster headache. In the case of common migraine and migraine equivalents, an inherent periodicity is less common, and the clinical pattern of attacks tends to be far more dependent on the external or emotional circumstances of the patient.

Duration Between Attacks

The length of time between successive attacks of classical migraine is usually somewhere between two and ten weeks, individual patients generally adhering fairly closely to their own time-patterns. Liveing cites the following figures:

[Of 35 patients with periodic migraine] in 9 cases the attacks returned once in a fortnight, and in 12 once a month; while intervals of 2 to 3 months prevailed in 7. The remaining 7 comprised exceptionally long or short periods.

Comparable figures were found by Klee (1968) in his series of 150 carefully documented cases, 33 percent of patients having migraines at intervals of less than 1 month, 20 percent of patients having migraines at intervals of 4 to 8 weeks, 26 percent at intervals of 8 to 12 weeks, and the remaining 21 percent at intervals of 3 months or more. My own experience of the incidence patterns of classical migraine is in accordance with these findings. It must be stressed, however, that crude incidence figures of this type may be ambiguous or even meaningless, unless care has been taken to exclude the effects of periodically recurring external or emotional circumstances provocative of migraines: we will later make reference to some determinants of a "pseudoperiodicity" of this type.

The grouping of common migraines, if the effects of adventitious circumstances can be excluded, tends to be more closely packed than that of classical migraines. A number of severely affected patients may have two or more attacks weekly, a frequency which would be most unusual in the case of classical migraine. We may note, in passing, that very frequent periodic common migraines show a striking tendency toward nocturnal occurrence. Patients who experience periodic common migraines only once a month (as in du Bois Reymond's case, quoted at the start of the first chapter) may often account themselves relatively lucky. Often but not always, for there appears to be a tendency toward a reciprocal relation between the frequency and the severity of such attacks, widely spaced attacks being correspondingly more severe. One of Liveing's patients expressed this concisely, and with a certain moral undertone, writing:

I have long ceased to care for longer intervals; I know that I have a *certain quantity of suffering* which I must go through, however it is broken up or divided, and I would as soon have it regularly as not.*

We may also consider cluster headache as a form of periodic migraine, provided that we regard the entire cluster (which may comprise a hundred individual attacks of migrainous neuralgia) as a single monstrous attack of migraine. The interval between clusters is far longer than that between common and classical migraines: an average interval might be a year, and the range of intervals will lie between three months and five years. Some clusters, it may be added, occur at annual intervals almost to the day.

Bizarre patterns of intermittency are sometimes seen, as in the following case, unique in my experience, which shows periodic clustering of common migraines:

Case 52

A 55-year-old man of serene disposition who has experienced annual "sieges" of common migraine for nineteen years. For a period of four to six weeks, he is utterly incapacitated by almost daily attacks of great severity and considerable duration (twelve to twenty hours). These attacks are characterized by bilateral vascular headache, intense nausea, repeated vomiting, and many other autonomic symptoms, that is to say, in no sense resembling attacks of migrainous neuralgia. The siege begins and ends suddenly, for no apparent reason, and the patient is wholly exempt from migraine for the remainder of the year.

The most irregular patterns of occurrence are seen in some cases of classical migraine, and especially of isolated migraine auras. I have had a number of such patients who may have gone for six, twelve or thirty months without an attack, only to have a sudden "bad period" with three to four attacks in quick succession.

---

*Similar sentiments are often expressed by patients with manic-depressive cycles. Such cycles represent not only physiological and chemical alterations in the body, but *moral cycles* also, with exemption from the harsher dictates of conscience during periods of elation, and an exaggeration of conscience in the self-hating, self-accusing periods of depression. The depression is often felt to be payment for the mania, as a vicious migraine may be anticipated after a protracted exemption from pain.

Immunity Between Attacks

There is, characteristically, a time of absolute immunity to further attack following every severe attack of periodic migraine, as du Bois Reymond has reminded us:*

For a certain period after the attack I can expose myself with impunity to influences which before would have infallibly produced an attack.

The immunity diminishes by degrees, and the likelihood of the next attack increases commensurately. Following the termination of absolute immunity, gross provocations may elicit a (somewhat premature) attack. As the relative immunity grows less, more and more trifling stimuli may suffice to detonate the impending attack. Finally, when the attack is "due" (or a little overdue), it *will* occur, explosively, whether or not there is any provocation.

Essentially similar cycles of sensitivity and immunity to attack are seen in many cases of idiopathic epilepsy and asthma. In each case, on a different time scale, one must envisage the same form of graduated refractoriness and sudden discharge which is characteristic of all biological cycles, from the millisecond intermittency of nerve-impulses to the annual sheddings of leaves and skins.

Approach of the Attack

Periodic migraines, more clearly than others, especially if they are severe and infrequent, tend to have clear-cut prodromal symptoms, restlessness, irritability, constipation, water retention, and so on, before common or classical migraines, and sometimes a peculiar form of burning or local discomfort before the onset of a cluster attack (as in case 7). Patients with extremely infrequent, severe attacks may experience other forms of physiological premonition for some days before the actual attack, as tiny seismic disturbances may signal the approach of a major earthquake. Thus one patient (case

---

*Perhaps the most dramatic example of post-ictal immunity is seen with reference to cluster headache. During the cluster, patients may be exquisitely sensitive to the taking of alcohol; following the cluster, they can immediately take quantities of alcohol without ill-effects. The approach of a subsequent cluster may be signalled, before any spontaneous attacks of pain, by the recurrence of alcohol-sensitivity and mild alcohol-induced attacks.

16), who experienced attacks of classical migraine every year or two, observed luminous spots darting across his visual field for two to three days before each attack. Other patients may suffer from myoclonic jerks, chiefly at night, for a day or two before each rare attack, a symptom which is shared by some epileptics.

Pseudoperiodicity

We have set apart periodic migraines, somewhat arbitrarily, as expressions of an inherent cyclical process in the nervous system. In practice, we may encounter considerable difficulty in demarcating the effects of innate neuronal periodicity from those of other internal cycles (physiological or emotional) or of undiscovered external cycles. We may demonstrate these ambiguities by a few clinical examples.

A colleague of mine, who suffers from migrainous neuralgia, affirms that his attacks wake him at exactly three o'clock every morning, and that, if necessary, he could set his watch by this. Shall we ascribe such attacks to some idiosyncratic Circadian cycle in his nervous system, to some occult physiological cycle elsewhere in the body, to the chiming of a distant clock causing a migrainous conditioned reflex, or to some dark childhood memory (the witnessing of a primal scene) associated with this dangerous hour? A patient of mine (case 10), who has been subject for many years to monthly attacks of classical migraine, occasionally replaced by abdominal migraine or violent mood disturbance, insisted that his attacks always coincided with a full moon, and produced a remarkable diary in support of this. When he gave me his history, I recalled the old words of Willis, about "the great aspects of the sun and moon" as determinants of migraine. The patient appeared obsessed by his lunar migraines, but whether the moon caused the migraine, and the migraine the obsession, or whether the obsession caused the migraine, I could not distinguish. An uncanny periodicity may also characterize "anniversary migraines" which are analogous to anniversary neuroses. I think, in this context, of one patient, a nun, who professed to have a classical migraine every Good Friday, a contemporary version of Easter stigmata. Personal anniversaries—of birthdays, marriages, disasters and traumas, and so forth—not in-

frequently determine strictly periodic attacks of migraine, or of
other functional illnesses.

One of the recurring themes of this book is that migraines are
enacted at many simultaneous levels, and that their machinery,
similarly, may be set in motion at any or every level. Although the
precipitant of periodic, idiopathic migraines is, by definition, a
neuronal one, we must allow that equally effective trigger
mechanisms may exist at many other levels, from local segmental
reflexes which have assumed a ticlike sensitivity, to recurrent
stimuli at the highest level, in the forms of obsessive expectations,
recapitulative fantasies, and the like. Whether the clockwork is
originally at a cellular level (as in allergic reactions), at a molecular
level, at the level of cerebral periodicities, or at the level of motive
and emotion, may subsequently become irrelevant, for the periodicity of the attacks may finally become immanent and *entrenched* at
every functional level. Such considerations suggest themselves with
particular force in the interpretation of menstrual migraines, in
which it is most useful to regard the migraine, not as a response to
a single isolated "factor," but as a reflector of many simultaneous
periodicities—of hormone level, of fundamental physiological and
biological periodicities, *and* of concurrent moods and motives. Any
one of these, one may suspect, may on occasion perpetuate the
periodic pattern, as is implied in the following history:

Case 74

This 68-year-old woman had experienced menstrual migraines, and no
others, since the age of 21. Her menopause, thirty years later, made no
difference to the pattern, her attacks continuing to occur at twenty-eight
to thirty day intervals.

Conclusions

The forms of migraine considered in this chapter illustrate, *par
excellence*, the Willisian notion of "idiopathy," sudden explosions
set off in a charged and waiting nervous system. Liveing's term
"nervestorms" is an incomparable metaphor, for one cannot avoid
visualizing the slow gathering of forces and tensions in the nervous

system, the sudden breaking of an electrical storm, the ensuing serenity and clear skies.*

In attacks of this type, the entire migraine—from the first coruscation of the aura, or first intimation of prodromal excitation, to the last echoes following the resolution of the attack—presents itself as an integral unit; it is, so to speak, preformed and complete, with an irresistible tendency to move through its course until it dies away and permits the establishment of a new (if temporary) physiological equilibrium. Periodic and paroxysmal migraines are difficult to avert and difficult to abort, but in return promise an ensuing immunity of substantial length. They also tend, in their symptoms and styles, to be the most stereotyped of all migraines, the least tailored to circumstantial considerations, and the least flavored with emotional undertones and strategies. They are *precipitated*, abruptly and completely, from physiological solution, in a manner reminiscent of a sudden crystallization from a supersaturated solution. They mark the climax and ending of a physiological season; the attack is *dehisced*, like the bursting of ripe fruit, so that the cycle may start into motion again.

*Liveing explicitly distinguishes the notion of nerve force from that of the accumulation of any *substance*. His conception is a purely physiological one:

"a gradually increasing instability of equilibrium in the nervous parts: when this reaches a certain point, the balance of forces is liable to be upset and the train of paroxysmal phenomena determined by causes in themselves totally inadequate to produce such effects—just as a mere scratch will shiver to dust a mass of unannealed glass. . . ."

He comes to this conclusion from a consideration of the enormous number of factors of different kinds which can precipitate an attack:

"the impression may come from without, and be of the nature of an irritation of some peripheral nerve, visceral, muscular, or cutaneous; or it may reach the centers through the circulation . . . or it may descend from the higher centres of physical activity. . . ."

So many exciting factors, yet the effect is the same: in every case the nervous system responds with a migraine. Therefore, the migraine is *implicit* in the cerebral repertoire. Its structure is, as it were, *preformed*.

8

Circumstantial Migraine

We will be concerned, in this chapter, with the consideration of circumstances which tend to provoke attacks of migraine. We will confine our terms of reference to *acute, transient states* which, as such, may elicit a single attack of migraine, while deferring discussion of chronic circumstantial provocation to the following chapter. Our data are culled, for the most part, from the observations of reliable patients who have learned to watch the occurrence of their own attacks, to keep diaries, and act as impartial observers of their own propensities. These data are supplemented, here and there, by experimental observations made under controlled conditions. We must reiterate, yet again, that one cannot hope to establish a one-to-one relation between circumstance and attack; there is at most a general tendency between the two.

The circumstances which we have to consider are so various and so numerous, that some form of preliminary classification is necessary as an aid to exposition. The categories adopted are purely informal and pretend to no rigor.

AROUSAL MIGRAINES

This term denotes the occurrence of migraines in circumstances which activate, arouse, annoy, and jangle the organism.* Among

---

*A similar miscellany of arousing circumstances may provoke many analogous reactions as, for example, hay fever. As Sydney Smith remarked of himself in this connection: "The membrane is so irritable, that light, dust, contradiction, an absurd remark, the sight of a dissenter, anything, sets me a-sneezing."

such circumstances we may recognize the following: light, noise, smells, inclement climate, exercise, excitement, violent emotion, somatic pain, and the action of certain drugs. We should also include in this category, as *intrinsic* excitations liable to be followed by a migraine reaction, the arousal of migrainous prodromes, and auras. This list makes no pretense of being complete.

Light and Noise

There are many patients who insist that glaring light and blaring noise are liable to give them a migraine. Emphasis is usually laid upon the intensity and duration of the provocative circumstance, upon its unbearability, upon the annoyance which precedes the attack, and the explicit wish to terminate the experience and find quiet and modest illumination. A number of patients in this class enter one's consulting room wearing dark glasses, and not a few of them have learned the word "photophobic." Crowded summer beaches with sunlight beating down upon the ocean, and machine shops blazing with unshielded lights, are common grounds of complaint. Other patients claim specific intolerance of films and television.

With regard to the last of these, the question of *flickering light* as a highly specific provocative circumstance must be considered. The presumed mechanism of reaction in such cases is a special one, and will be discussed separately later in this chapter.

Smells

We have noted the occasional occurrence of olfactory hallucinations in migraine aura, and the rather common enhancement, distortion and intolerance of smells which may occur *during* a migraine: both of these, no doubt, are responsible for a number of spurious or misleading histories which would otherwise seem to inculpate smells as a provocative circumstance. Yet there do exist, additional to these, reliable patients who appear to have developed, or possess innately, a specific sensitivity to certain smells (tar is often mentioned), or a general sensitivity to "bad" smells. Such histories are particularly common in the colorful older literature. Liveing, for example, cites the case of the following patient:

a distinguished member of the Academy, and a hospital physician, who cannot take part in a post-mortem examination without being instantly seized by vomiting and an attack of migraine. The same thing happens if by any chance they omit thoroughly to ventilate the wards which are under his care before his visit.*

Inclement Weather

Any or all climatic extremes, it would seem, may occasion an attack of migraine in suitably predisposed patients, or be blamed for doing so. Storms and winds are the classical examples, and there are a number of patients who claim a sort of meteorological clairvoyance, and avow that they can predict the approach of the Hamsin or Santa Ana, or of impending thunder, from the migraines they suffer at such times. A colleague of mine tells me that her Swiss childhood was marred, at certain times, by migraines which occurred during the annual southwesterly gales which blow across Zürich, and that she never suffered attacks at any other time.

Other patients, less exotic in their reactions, tend to have repeated migraines in very hot or humid weather. Here the provocative circumstances should perhaps be construed differently, as likely to induce listlessness and prostrated states which favor the appearance of migraine.

Exercise, Excitement, Emotion

Violent exercise (which must in its nature include elements of both physiological and psychological excitement) is often mentioned as a unique occasion of migraine by younger patients. Characteristically, the attack comes on shortly *after* the exercise, very rarely during it. We may recall a patient cited earlier (case 25) whose classical-cumfacioplegic attacks would come after a violently competitive cross-country race, and at no other time.

*We must make an observation, in this context, which may be applied willy-nilly to many of the odder and more idiosyncratic circumstances sometimes held responsible for migraine attacks, that is to say that a true organic sensitivity may be mimicked by what Liveing would call a "pathological habit," namely a conditioned reflex. We may remember such patients with "rose fever" who start to sneeze if presented with a paper rose.

Violent emotions exceed all other acute circumstances in their capacity to provoke migraine reactions, and in many patients—especially sufferers from classical migraine—are responsible for the vast majority of all attacks experienced. Liveing writes: "It does not seem to matter much what the character of the emotion is, provided it be strongly felt." I think, however, that we can be more specific: we find, in practice, that sudden *rage* is the commonest precipitant, although *fright* (panic) may be equally potent in younger patients. Sudden *elation* (at a moment of triumph or unexpected good fortune) may have the same effect.

Such reactions have a paradoxical quality, in that they tend to *arrest* a person in midexcitement, or immediately following the peak of excitement. There are a variety of clinical parallels, some of which can serve as "alternatives" to the migraine reaction: we must particularly note the extremely acute reactions of narcolepsy and cataplexy (which frequently occur in response to rage, orgasm, or hilarious excitement), the reactions of "fainting" (vasovagal syncope) and "swooning" (hysterical stupor) in response to a sudden emotional "shock"—pleasant or unpleasant—and, in more pathological contexts, the reactions of "freezing" (as exhibited by Parkinsonian patients) and "blocking" (as exhibited by schizophrenic patients). Nor are reactions of this type confined to human beings: we will find reference to a variety of biological analogues and homologues in Part III.

It should be observed that the provocative emotions in all cases would be ranked as "kinetic" in James Joyce's terminology: they arouse the organism and tend in their normal course to lead to action (fight, flight, jumping for joy, laughing, etc.). They may be contrasted with the "static" emotions (dread, horror, pity, awe, etc.) which are expressed in stillness and silence, and slowly abate, after many hours, by lysis or catharsis. It is exceedingly rare for such static emotions to ignite a migraine.

We may recognize here two *styles* of dissipating tension or emotion: the ejaculation (whether this be verbal, somatic or visceral) which suddenly dissipates a state of tension; and a slow leaking away, a lysis, which accomplishes the same end more gradually: laughter versus tears, the spark versus the corposant.

Other forms of psychophysiological excitement may be mentioned briefly. A few patients are unfortunate enough to experience migraines immediately following *orgasm*: see case 2 and case 55.

Finally, as we have already intimated, the entire cycle of excitation/inhibition may become integral and internalized, an aura or prodrome acting as provocation for a migraine.

Pain

Somatic pain (from muscle and skin) tends to provoke and arouse; visceral pain (from viscera, vessels, etc.) tends to have the opposite effect, to produce nausea, passivity, and so on. Both may induce migraines, although by different mechanisms. Perhaps the commonest example of the former in action is provided by the occurrence of an acute (muscle) injury in an active man, who, aroused, enraged and thwarted by the pain, develops a migraine superimposed upon his other problems. The effects of visceral pain will be considered subsequently.

The question of *drug actions* in relation to migraine will be relegated to a separate discussion later in this chapter.

SLUMP MIGRAINES AND CRASH REACTIONS

These neologisms denote the occurrence of migraines in circumstances of exhaustion, prostration, sedation, passivity, sleep, and so forth. Many of these circumstances are normally and physiologically associated with states of pleasant satiety and consummation, delectable drowsiness and lassitude, and healing sleep. But let the physiological reaction be more intense, let it assume an unpleasing affective tone, and we see a *slump reaction* of one type or another. Slump reactions thus represent exaggerations and travesties of peaceful and restful states.

Eating and Fasting

A hearty meal is followed by pleasant feelings of satisfaction and consummation, a little doziness, and the active, but inconspicuous, processes of digestion, and the like. A closer scrutiny will reveal a multiplicity of postprandial reactions:

The picture has been presented of parasympathetic activity in an old man sleeping after dinner. His heart rate is slow, his breathing noisy because of bronchial constriction; his pupils are small; drops of saliva may run out of the corner of his mouth. A stethoscope applied to his abdomen will reveal much intestinal activity [Burn, 1963].

This description provides an unappetizing, almost a Swiftian, dissection of a dear old man enjoying his after-dinner nap.

Now consider these same physiological reactions amplified, distorted, and rendered symptomatic. We may recognize three slump-syndromes in this regard: "indigestion," "dumping syndrome," and "postprandial migraine." We may say, if we wish, that the first is "due" to an overloaded stomach, and the second to acute hypoglycemia—although both contentions are questionable. Phenomenologically, however, they all represent parodies, or pathological variations of normal postprandial torpor and vegetative state.

We must also consider certain pathological reactions to *fasting*. When some hours have elapsed since a meal, the "normal" reaction is to become somewhat restless and wonder when dinner is due, namely appetite activity and arousal. If no meal is forthcoming and the fast extended, there will sooner or later supervene symptoms of prostration or collapse. In a few patients the blood sugar will fail to be maintained after x hours of fasting. And a small but definite proportion of patients are liable to migraine reactions under these circumstances.

Case 54

This 47-year-old woman experienced three to five common migraines a month with no immediately discernible cause for these. She was instructed to keep a diary, in the hope that this might uncover some provocative circumstances not previously attended to. Her diary revealed, on her next clinic visit, that her attacks tended to come if she missed breakfast. An extended glucose tolerance-test was undertaken, which revealed a five-hour blood sugar of 44 mg percent. At this point the patient was pale, sweating, and complaining of headache. Further tests established the diagnosis of "functional hypoglycemia." The patient was instructed to make a point of having breakfast, and to keep sugared orange juice on her bedside table. Thereafter, she was virtually free of attacks.

Hot Weather and Fever

Normal reactions to hot weather include lassitude and sweating; when fever is present, malaise and vascular headache may be added to these symptoms. A number of migraine patients show over-reaction to thermal stimuli, and tend to get attacks in association with hot weather or fevers. Thus an attack of mild flu, or a febrile "cold" which would be trivial to a majority of people, may become the occasion of an incapacitating migraine in predisposed patients.

Passive Motion

Gentle passive motion is normally soothing and soporific—hence a baby may be rocked to sleep. In a certain portion of the population, however, the response to passive motion (or direct vestibular stimulation) is inordinate and intolerable—such people may suffer from intense "motion-sickness" in childhood (with nausea, vomiting, pallor, cold sweating, etc.) or thereafter; if vascular headache is present in addition to the above symptoms, a motion migraine will result. Exaggerated responses to vestibular stimulation is perhaps the commonest, and certainly one of the most incapacitating, idiosyncrasies of many migraine patients, and as such they may be shut off from many of the simpler pleasures in life: swings in childhood, roller coasters in adolescence, and travelling by bus, train, ship or plane at all times. It is important to note that *passivity* and passive stimulation are essential in these reactions; many patients who are extravagantly prone to motion-sickness are perfectly able to drive their own cars, or pilot their own boats and planes.

Exhaustion

A hard day's work normally leads to a delicious tiredness, but may, in predisposed patients, determine a pathological variant of this, namely exhaustion, incipient collapse, and sometimes migraine. There may be a similar incapacity to tolerate a loss of sleep which would readily be borne by the majority of the population. Such sleep deprivation is very likely to provoke a migraine or migranoid reaction in predisposed patients, and not infrequently other allied reactions discussed in chapter 5, particularly narcolepsy. Other factors, for example, illness, diarrhea, fasting, may summate with an otherwise inconsiderable fatigue or sleep deficit to a crucial level of exhaustion, at which point a slump reaction is likely to occur. Thus Parry (a sufferer from isolated visual auras) noted of himself that:

Violent fatigue, more especially when accompanied by from eight to ten hours' fasting . . . sometimes brings them on . . . so too has the exhaustion following a smart attack of diarrhea.

Drug Reactions

We have already touched on the subject of drug reactions in relation to migraine in various contexts, in allusion to "hangovers," abnormal reserpine reactions, and others. These too must be construed as exaggerations and perversions of normal physiological responses. Anyone is likely to feel sleepy, or slightly ill, after many drinks, but intense nausea, or a common migraine, or an attack of migrainous neuralgia after a single drink is excessive, and represents the abnormal reactivity many migraine patients must learn to accept in themselves, whether they choose to compromise with this predisposition, defy it, or "take a chance" on it. Similarly "hangovers," when florid, represent a pathological reactivity, and are not infrequently the harbinger, or first sign, of a future migraine candidate.

There are an immense number of depressant drugs besides alcohol, some of which are notoriously unsafe for certain patients. The most infamous of these is perhaps *reserpine*, which may be used, in a variety of proprietary preparations, to control hypertension. Reserpine may provoke not only migraine, but many other allied reactions, for example, stupor, narcolepsy, shock, (psychological) depression, and Parkinsonian akinesia.

The uses and abuses of the *amphetamines* must also be noted in this context. Amphetamines cause a powerful arousal of central and peripheral nervous activity, which is liable to be followed by a commensurate "slump" as their action wears off. We have already seen that some patients may make spontaneous comparisons of the excitatory; and inhibitory phases of their auras with amphetamine action(s) (see cases 67 and 69), and we will later have occasion to speak of the therapeutic uses of the amphetamines in migraine (Part

IV). Our concern at this stage is with the liability to migraine, and other allied reactions, in the "let-down" period after heavy amphetamine dosage. The following case history is instructive:

Case 43

This 23-year-old patient had been subject to one or two common migraines a month since the age of 19. Eight weeks before she consulted me, her condition had taken a sudden change for the worse. She described herself as now experiencing daily migraines, which at first were confluent with one another ("migraine status"). Other very recent symptoms included intense tiredness, frequent narcolepsies, persistent lacrimation, diarrhea, and depression. I was initially at a loss to explain this sudden and mysterious change in her state, and wondered whether some emotional tragedy had occurred of which she was reluctant to speak. On her second visit, she admitted that she had been addicted to Ritalin, and had been taking no less than 1,600 mg daily for over a year. When she stopped taking the drug abruptly, she experienced the above monstrous withdrawal syndrome of a depressive, slumped, parasympathetic "status."

Food, Migraine, and the Stomach

There is a sizable proportion of patients who, feeling ill ("bilious" or "dyspeptic") during or before the headache, ascribe all their attacks to "something I ate." In saying this, they unwittingly echo a long and ancient tradition of thought. This tradition may be exemplified by the following passage taken from Tissot's *Treatise*:

All patients remark that their stomachs are not as comfortable as usual on the approach of an attack; that if they are careful over them the attacks are not so frequent; and that if they take anything which deranges the stomach the attacks are more frequent and severe.

Persons who suffer from migraine and stomach derangement feel the migraine diminish in proportion as the stomach recovers itself. . . . Almost invariably, on the instant the stomach discharges its contents, the pains cease . . .

We will hold back Tissot's conclusions from his observations till the end of this chapter. Some of these clinical observations cannot be doubted; the difficulties lie in their interpretation. That gastric disorder may be *associated* with migraine or headache does not necessarily indicate that it is its cause.

The matter can be (and has in the past been) argued to and fro interminably. For myself, I regard any concomitant or antecedent "stomach derangement" as an integral part of the migraine composite. Further, though I cannot gainsay the observations of a patient who insists that his migraines come after eating ham or chocolate, and under no other circumstances, I must regard the interpretation of this empirical fact as exceptionally tricky. I am not convinced that a migraine can ever be ascribed to a specific food sensitivity, and I would suspect any association of the two to the establishment of a conditioned reflex.

"Chinese Restaurant Syndrome" and Other Migrainogenic Food

Experience since the first edition of this book has made clear that there *can be* specific food reactions, and that these may have a clearly defined chemical mechanism.

The phrase "Chinese restaurant syndrome" has become very familiar (though very distressing to Chinese restaurants!). Many persons, and an especially high proportion of migraineurs may show severe reactions to Chinese meals. In milder cases, there is just a feeling of malaise, with some shivering, pallor, borborygmus and nausea; in more severe cases there may be absolute prostration, with severe visceral and vascular upset (including a typical vascular headache), a confused and even delirious mental state and considerable faintness, if not actual "fainting." It is clear that such reactions come in the "borderlands" of migraine, and resemble the "migranoid reactions," the vasovagal attacks, the nitritoid crises, and so on described in chapter 2. It is evident that one is seeing a parasympathetic or "vagotonic" response—and one to which migraineurs are especially prone. It is not every Chinese meal (most fortunately!) which provokes this—and there was a delay of several years in recognizing that there was, indeed, a syndrome, because of its erratic and unpredictable occurrence. It took several years to incriminate the pathogenic factor—and when this was done it was found to be monosodium glutamate (MSG), very widely used as a food-additive for the enhancement of flavors, and by no means confined to Chinese restaurants (MSG, indeed, is not "natural" at all—and even in soy sauce is an artificial addition). A certain conflict of interests has arisen—as with so many potentially toxic additives: for MSG is uniquely useful as a flavor enhancer, and a majority of people will tolerate it well enough. However, with increased consciousness of its toxic potential, its use is less widespread and gross than it was before the syndrome was recognized about ten years ago.

Some migraineurs may find that there are certain other foods to which they are particularly sensitive—this is commonly remarked of strong *cheese*. Cheese (and several other foods) had indeed been regarded, back in the fifties, as carrying a specific danger for certain groups of patients—namely those receiving antidepressant drugs of the monoamine oxidase (MAO) inhibitor type: in such patients cheese and other foods might provoke a sudden and dangerous rise in blood pressure, and other autonomic effects—and it was partly for this reason that these drugs, extraordinarily affective as they were as antidepressants, gave way to the much safer, but (on the whole) less potent "tricyclics." The pathogenic factor here is *amines* of various sorts, especially *tyramine*, but others as well, which innocuous in themselves may activate (or be activated by) other chemical substances to produce stronger disturbances in the chemical control-systems of the brain, especially those concerned with autonomic control. Although migraineurs are not at *dangerous* risk (like patients taking MAO-inhibitors), they tend to have less latitude than the nonmigraineur.

One should make such a statement only to qualify it; it is not all migraineurs who show MSG intolerance, cheese intolerance, and so forth, but only *some*: and sometimes, indeed, for only some of the time. Such specificity and selectivity suggest that not all migraineurs are the same; that there may, for example, be several different subgroups, who may be distinguished on the basis of differing brain chemistries, so that some are upset (or helped) by a food substance or drug to which other migraineurs are more or less indifferent. Such considerations of chemical specificity, which are of no less practical than theoretical importance, will be further discussed in the latter sections of this book.

"Letdown" Situations

It is common knowledge that migraines tend to come "after the event," whatever the "event" is. Thus, patients often complain of experiencing migraines after an examination, a childbirth, a business triumph, a holiday, or other occurrences. An important recurrent pattern of this type is exemplified by "weekend migraines" (sometimes alternating with weekend depressions, diarrhea, "colds," etc.), during the slump-period which follows a hectic week. Such propensities will be discussed in greater detail in chapter 9, and in Part III.

Nocturnal Migraine

It is often a matter of astonishment to patients that they should sometimes be woken from sleep by a migraine, and their astonishment may only be increased when they are assured that an association between sleep and migraine is not merely common, but to be expected.

We may distinguish several varieties of nocturnal migraine on the basis of careful histories: there are attacks which come at the dead of night, jerking patients from the deepest sleep; there are attacks which tend to come at dawn, intruding on an uneasy half-waking slumber; there are attacks coalesced with dreams (the most reliable histories are obtained from some patients with classical migraine, who wake in the second or headache stage with a clear memory of dream images and scotomatous figures mixed together); and there are attacks associated with nightmares (night terrors and somnambulisms).

Attacks of migrainous neuralgia, *par excellence*, tend to wake patients from the deepest layers of sleep. The onset of such attacks is extremely acute, yet those who experience nocturnal attacks are never able to recollect any dreams from the time of their onset.

Classical migraine is sometimes nocturnal, and common migraine is very frequently so; I have notes of more than forty severely affected patients whose many attacks were *exclusively* nocturnal. Many such patients assert that they dream more, or more vividly, on nights when they suffer migraines, and all-night electroencephalographic studies performed on some such patients have shown an apparent increase in the amount of paradoxical (rapid eye-movement, or dreaming) sleep associated with their attacks (Dr. J. Dexter, 1968: personal communication).

Exceptionally clear histories are given by nightmare-prone patients regarding the frequent linking together of the nightmare experience and subsequent migraine symptoms (see case 75, for example). The fact of the association is clearer than its interpretation; it is difficult to assert whether the dreaming or nightmare experience causes a migraine, is caused by a migraine, or simply shows a number of clinical and physiological similarities to the migraine experience.

Nor indeed are these interpretations mutually exclusive. We have cited a number of case histories illustrating the occurrence of "dreamy states," delirious states and "daymares" as components of migraine auras, and one may question whether in some cases of very constant conjunction between nightmares and classical migraines, the former is not itself the chief or sole manifestation of an aura.

Equally plausibly, one may conceive the intense emotional and physiological excitation of the dreaming (and especially the nightmare) state to provide an adequate arousal stimulus for migraines in predisposed subjects. One can do no more, at the present time, than note the undoubted affinity of migraines to occur during sleep, and to be associated, in particular, with restless and dreaming sleep.

RESONANCE MIGRAINE

We must consider under this head one important, highly specific, if somewhat rare, form of circumstantial migraine, namely the elicitation of a scintillating scotoma by flickering light of certain frequencies, patterned visual stimuli of specific type, and even certain visual images and memories.*

Flickering light from any source—emitted from a fluorescent or television tube, reflecting from cinema screens or metallic surfaces, and so on—may elicit the *immediate* appearance of a scintillating

*A charming example of an aural response to visually patterned and intermittent stimulation is provided by a case history cited in Liveing, in which the patient's attacks were evoked by the sight of falling snow, and no other circumstance.

scotoma with a scintillation rate identical with the frequency of the provocative stimulus. The use of a stroboscope demonstrates that only flicker frequencies in a narrow band (between eight to twelve stimuli per second) are effective in provoking the scintillating scotoma. The same frequency band has also been shown to be most effective in provoking photo-myoclonic jerking or true photo-epilepsy in predisposed patients.

I have received accurate descriptions of such photogenic scotomata from several patients, one of the most interesting of these being a nurse who also exhibited photomyoclonus and photoepilepsy as alternative responses to flickering light.

A visual fixation on appropriate patterns may similarly serve as flickering stimuli. Several descriptions of this are provided by Liveing:

M. Piorry says of himself . . . that he can produce the phenomenon of the luminous vibratory circle at will by strongly fixing the sight, or reading.

Reference is also made to a patient whose attacks had occasionally been brought on by looking at a striped wallpaper or a striped dress. We must recognize the closest analogy between these phenomena and those of photoepilepsy and reading-epilepsy. In the case of the former, for example, a moving patterned stimulus may be provided by rapidly waving the fingers before the eyes, or—in one published case—bobbing up and down before a venetian blind.

The analogy may be pressed even further. Penfield and Perot (1963), in a massive review of their epileptic patients, describe the "psychical precipitation" of attacks in some patients by vivid visualization of the circumstances of the original (primal) attack. Similarly it is noted by Liveing concerning Sir John Herschel "a sufferer from purely visual megrim states . . . that an attack was produced in him by allowing the mind to dwell on the description of the appearances."

We are forced to seek an explanation for two facts: the *immediacy* of the scotomatous response, and its numerically precise *synchronization* with the flicker stimulus. The most economical conjecture is that such phenomena are due to a quantitative attunement, or *resonance* within the nervous system, following the impact of appropriate stimuli.

Addendum

The provocative stimuli are not necessarily visual—the very word "resonance" is suggestive of sound! Intolerance of noise (phonophobia) is an almost universal feature of the irritability characteristic of many migraines (see p. 27), but what needs emphasis here is the *peculiarly* aggravating, or provocative power of *sounds of certain frequencies*.

We live in an increasingly assaultive and noisy environment, and one may obtain the clearest histories of the provocative effects of this in some migraineurs. Some patients are immediately affected by the sound of pneumatic drills—and speak of the rapid, repetitive chattering of these as being peculiarly provocative of migraines—not just their intensity, but the *chatter* of their noise. The combination of high intensity with insistent repetition makes the beat of loud rock music migrainogenic to some patients, a phenomenon analogous to musicogenic epilepsy.

That it is not the intensity of the sound as such; nor some particular hated timbre, but, very specifically, its *frequency* that is intolerable, may be tested experimentally in a clinical laboratory, monitoring the patient's brain waves by EEG. One may find, in these circumstances, that it is only *particular frequencies* of flashing light or banging noise which cause gross disturbance in the brain wave patterns, *driving* these first, in synchrony with the stimulus, and then *kindling* a severe, paroxysmal cerebral response.

In striking contrast, pleasant, melodious and truly musical stimuli rapidly restore constancy and rhythmicity to the brain waves, and terminate the paroxysmal response, both clinically and electrically. We may see very clearly how the *wrong* sound, or "anti-music," *is* pathogenic and migrainogenic; while the *right* sound—proper music—is truly tranquillizing, and immediately restores cerebral health. These effects are striking, and quite fundamental, and put one in mind of Novalis' aphorism: "Every disease is a musical problem; every cure is a musical solution."

A similar response—first "driving," then "kindling" (to use key words in the electroencephalographic parlance)—may be evoked by *tactile stimuli*. A nice example of this was given in chapter 3 (case 75), where the intense vibrato of a motorbike was provocative of a migraine.

MIGRAINES PROVOKED BY VISUAL
FIELD DISTORTIONS

As migraines may be evoked by unusual rhythms and disturbances in *time*, so may they be provoked by odd symmetries or asymmetries in *space*. The following history from a gifted observer (case 77) indicates this strange spatial sensitivity or vulnerability in some patients:

As some of my migraines start with disturbances in my visual field, so some may be *provoked* by unexpected twists and oddities which suddenly strike me. A button may be done up askew in a coat. The whole coat looks askew and bothers me oddly. Then this skew in the coat *becomes* a skew or twist in my vision, sets off a local distortion in my visual field, which may then spread until it engulfs the greater part of the visual field. Or it may be something askew in a face—like a tic, or a grimace, or a spasm—some asymmetry. Once it was set off by seeing a man with Bell's Palsy. The perception is momentary, but it can set off a spatial disturbance that lasts for several minutes.

Klee speaks of strange forms of "metamorphopsia"—distortion of contours, eccentric misplacements within the visual field, micropsia, macropsia, and the like—as occurring in severe migraine auras (see p. 87), but does not discuss the *induction* of visual auras, in some patients, by the altered or unexpected appearances of things. The migraineur—like the artist—may be singularly sensitive to any "transformations," deformations, or divergences from the expected. They may induce for him a spreading topological deformation, a whole topsy-turvy, Escher-like, world of strange distortion. Once this is *recognized* by the patient, it ceases to be a bewilderment or terror, and can become—as perhaps it was for Escher—a stimulus to the creative imagination.

MISCELLANEOUS CIRCUMSTANTIAL MIGRAINES

We have by no means exhausted our listing of the circumstances under which migraines tend to occur, but we face serious difficulties in attempting to categorize what remains. We must deal with the following topics: migraine in relation to the bowels, especially constipation; in relation to menstrual periods, and hormones; and in relation to allergies. We will conclude with a brief consideration of "sympathetic" migraine, in relation to the above concomitances and certain other aspects of the attack itself.

The Bowels and Migraine

As some patients favor a gastric theory, so others are convinced of the intestinal origin of migraine, and have been moved to this conclusion by noting the association of their own migraines with disturbances of the bowel, particularly antecedent constipation. Here again, as with the question of stomach derangement and migraine, they are the unconscious heirs of a long tradition of belief. One may be given extraordinarily persuasive case histories, such as the following:

Case 4

A highly intelligent, not obviously moralistic or superstitious man of 28 who has suffered from migrainous neuralgia since childhood. He averages four to six attacks a month; there has never been either clustering or remission of attacks. This patient is emphatic that each attack is preceded by two or three days of constipation. For the remainder of the month, his bowels are regular and he is free from attacks. All the usual therapeutic approaches to migrainous neuralgia were tried and failed. Finally, with some embarassment, I placed the patient on regular laxatives. He went an unprecedented period of three months without either constipation or migraines.

What shall we say? That the constipation is, in fact, an integral portion of the migraine—its prodrome: that the stuffed bowel produces a factor which may lead to migraine: or that a conditioned reflex has been set in motion? Any of these might be the case; the likelihood is, migraine being so overdetermined a reaction, that *all* of them are the case.

MIGRAINE IN RELATION TO MENSTRUAL PERIODS AND HORMONES

We have already alluded (chapter 2) to the invariable occurrence of autonomic and affective disturbances at the menses, and the occurrence of outspoken menstrual migraines, at least occasionally, in 10 to 20 percent of all women during their reproductive periods. I have seen about 500 women with common migraines, and I would estimate that one-third of these experience menstrual migraines *in addition* to other attacks. I have notes of more than fifty patients who experience migraines *exclusively* at the menstrual periods. In contrast to these figures, the occurrence of classical migraine shows very much less tendency to be coupled with menstrual periods: of a total of fifty female patients with classical migraine, for example, only four have mentioned their occurrence at the menses, and none has experienced attacks confined to this time. Migrainous neuralgia is rare in women, and when it does occur, it appears to follow its own rhythm rather than the menstrual cycle.

Observations regarding the frequency of migraine at different times of the female life have been made since antiquity, and provide us with evidence of considerable consistency if questionable interpretation. We have emphasized the frequency of menstrual migraine, but we must note that attacks are by no means invariably premenstrual; a large minority of women experience attacks during and after the menstrual flow. We must note also that menstrual migraines, although they usually cease at the menopause, may in some cases continue to occur with the same periodicity after the menopause (see case 74). Much less common than menstrual migraines, but distinctive when they occur, are attacks experienced in the middle of the menstrual cycle, and presumed to be concomitant with ovulation. Common migraine is relatively rare before the onset of menstruation; classical migraine, however, shows no such restriction, and has frequently been recorded in early childhood. Very dramatic is the remission of migraine which may occur during pregnancy, characteristically during the latter half or last trimester of pregnancy; 80 to 90 percent of all women with common migraine are likely to experience such a remission during their first pregnancy, and a smaller number will secure relief in subsequent pregnancies; remission is much less striking in cases of classical migraine (but see case 11). Patients who have been exempt from migraine during the latter part of pregnancy not infrequently experience an exceptionally severe postpartum migraine one or two weeks after delivery. Finally, a matter of great contemporary concern, there are the varied and controversial effects of different hormone preparations—especially oral contraceptives—upon the severity and frequency of migraine attacks.

The subject is one of particular complexity, for the major changes in female reproductive function must be considered at so many levels: there are local changes in the uterus, and so on, there are specific hormonal changes, there are very general physiological changes (at puberty, at the menses, at the menopause), and, finally, there are important psychological concomitants of all these changes. Which of these, we must inquire, carries the greatest weight in determining patterns of migraine throughout life?

Classical physiology viewed menstrual migraines as a form of hysteria: thus Willis and Whytt envisaged these migraines as being generated by local changes in the uterus, their symptoms being radiated throughout the body by a direct organ-to-organ transmission or "sympathy." This notion of "uterine megrim" was still very generally held in the middle of the last century. Liveing considered all such theories of local origin in great detail, and found them inadequate to cover the known facts, concluding:

It is . . . to a widespread periodic excitation of the nervous system, and not to any mere uterine, or cerebral or general plethora pending the [menstrual] discharge, that I trace the manifestations of certain morbid tendencies on the part of the system, whether in the form of hysteria, megrim, epilepsy, or insanity, at these particular periods.

But Liveing knew nothing of hormones, and perhaps underestimated the ability of general physiological disturbances or psychological factors to modify a widespread periodic excitation of the nervous system.

It should not be difficult, one would imagine, to dissect out the role of hormonal influences, as opposed to other determinants, by observing the effect of purified hormonal preparations upon the severity and frequency of migraine attacks. There is, indeed, a vast literature on this topic, relating both to the effects of various hormone contraceptives on migraine patterns, and the effects of administering a variety of purified hormone preparations—androgens, estrogens, progestogens, gonadotrophins, and so forth.

The vastness of this literature (which has been repeatedly and carefully reviewed) is a measure of the difficulty which has been encountered in coming to any clear conclusions. Thus, it was postulated, from the occurrence of ovulatory and premenstrual migraines, that these attacks were precipitated, respectively, by raised levels of estrogen and by relatively sudden diminutions of circulating progestogens. Experience with current oral contraceptives has neither confirmed nor refuted this surmise: some contraceptives seemingly aggravate migraine, others appear to mitigate it, and yet others to have no effect upon migraine patterns; these varying effects have not been adequately correlated with the precise composition of the contraceptive used. Dramatic results have been claimed from the therapeutic use of androgens, estrogens, progestogens and gonadotrophins in the treatment of migraine: all such studies, however, have represented "straight" trials of the hormone, with the notorious ambiguities which attach to all such uncontrolled studies, particularly in regard to migraine which is infinitely placebo-sensitive (see chapter 14). One must deplore the publicity which often attaches to such studies, and the subsequent touting of unproven or even dangerous hormone preparations as cures for migraine.

The number of carefully controlled, double-blind trials of simple purified hormone preparations is exceedingly small. One may cite the recent study published by Bradley and others (1968) concerning the effects of fluorinated progesterone (Demigran) on migraine patients. Bradley and others found *no* significant effects upon the severity or frequency of migraine, save in the special case of menstrual attacks, which appeared to be slightly milder during Demigran administration.

There is a startling contrast between the modest or negative findings of such controlled studies and the spectacular results which have been claimed on the basis of "straight" trials of various hormone preparations. The entire subject is urgently in need of experimental clarification; certainly there is no strong evidence, at the present time, that any existing hormone preparation has *specific* (as opposed to placebo) therapeutic effects upon the occurrence of migraine.

One encounters, in practice, many case histories which suggest that other factors—particularly the patient's needs and expectations—may play an important part in determining the occurrence or disappearance of menstrual migraines, the remission of migraines during pregnancy, and the like. The following case history may be considered:

Case 31

A 32-year-old Catholic woman with severe menstrual migraines. She had had four children, the last of which required an exchange transfusion, in view of an Rh-incompatibility between the patient and her husband. Further pregnancies were considered undesirable, but the patient was constrained by her religious persuasions from taking any contraceptive measures. A gynecologist was consulted, who informed the patient that she had "abnormally high levels of estrogen" which were the cause of her menstrual migraines. He said that he would prescribe *for this* a hormone preparation (Ortho-Novum); he added that Ortho-Novum also happened to be a contraceptive, but its employment, in her case, was purely therapeutic, and only incidentally contraceptive. The patient's scruples were overcome by this assurance, and she consented to take the hormone. Her menstrual migraines vanished, and a year later had not returned.

This history is quoted, of course, for its ambiguity, not its simplicity. The effects of the hormone preparation were clear, but the interpretation of its effects are far from clear. It would seem eminently possible, in this case, that the patient, justifiably and chronically terrified of further pregnancies, was restored to emotional calm by the knowledge of the pill's contraceptive power, and that *this* was the crucial factor in curing her migraine. One sees many cases of menstrual migraines, indeed, which respond excellently to psychotherapy and this alone, suggesting that hormonal influences are at most a *codeterminant* of such migraine patterns. There is also considerable evidence that the remission of migraines during pregnancy is at least as dependent upon the patient's state of mind and attitudes to pregnancy as upon any alterations in hormonal balance (see, for example, case 56, cited in the following chapter).

We must conclude, therefore, that although menstruation, the menopause, and pregnancy, may have a profound effect in determining the patterns of migraine in certain patients, the mechanism of their action is uncertain, and is probably to be ascribed to multiple concomitant causes rather than the specific effects of hormonal changes.

Allergies and Migraine

We have already observed the high incidence of allergic reactions in migraine patients, and the postulate (put forward by Balyeat and many others) that migraines, when they occur in patients with multiple allergies, are themselves to be regarded as allergic reactions. But statistical correlation per se implies nothing beyond the fact of concomitance: it does not imply any logical or causal connection between the two phenomena which are being correlated.

But the belief that migraine may be allergic in basis is widespread, and many migraine patients, after migrating from one doctor to another, finally place themselves in the hands of an allergist. This is likely to be followed by the elaborate ritual of testing for "sensitivities" and following this, by a series of impressive rules and prohibitions—avoiding dusts and pollens, changing the bed linen, exiling the cat, eliminating all sorts of delectables from the diet, and other measures. This solemn regimen will be reinforced by frequent injections, designed to "desensitize" the patient. Not infrequently, a therapeutic triumph is achieved, or claimed.*

But neither statistical correlation nor therapeutic magic is evidence for an allergic basis. It is necessary, as with hormone trials, to investigate the matter with rigorous controls and techniques, as has been done by Wolff and many other workers (see Wolff, *Headache and Other Head Pain*, 1963, pp. 327–31) and such stringent approaches have indicated the extreme rarity of an allergic basis for migraines; less than one percent of all migraine attacks are explicable in terms of allergic sensitivities or mechanisms.

The frequent coexistence of migrainous and allergic reactions in many patients, and their occasional capacity to "replace" each other in response to particular provocative circumstances, is nevertheless remarkable, and requires explanation. We can only intimate our belief, at this stage, that migraine and allergic reactions are biologically *analogous*, and though fundamentally different in nature (allergic reactions representing local cellular sensitivities, and mi-

---

*There is, of course, a strong *moral* undertone to such regimens, as is true of so many successful ways of treating migraine. Sydney Smith, who suffered from hay fever, stresses the ascetic nature of his treatment: ". . . I am taking all proper care of myself, which care consists in eating nothing that I like, and doing nothing that I wish."

grainous reactions complex cerebral responses) may be employed in similar ways by a patient. This is essentially the conclusion reached by Wolff who has suggested that "the allergic disturbances and the migraine headache [may be] separate and independent manifestations of difficulty in adaptation."

Self-Perpetuation of Migraines

We cannot leave the subject of circumstantial migraines without asking ourselves two questions—questions which appear simple even to absurdity when formulated, but which are difficult to answer without bringing up concepts of a radical and even paradoxical kind. First, we must ask, why do migraines last *so long*? We remarked in the last chapter that periodic (idiopathic) attacks usually moved through a compact predetermined course, and are over; circumstantial migraines, on the contrary, have a tendency to prolong themselves, often for day after day, long past the original provocative circumstances. Second, we must ask, is it possible for one symptom or component of a migraine to have a *direct* action upon another one?

We spoke in the Historical Introduction, of the ancient "sympathetic" theories of migraine which dominated thinking for so many centuries, and we must now wonder whether any fragments of truth could have been caught up in the general framework of these theories, and, if so, whether they may be of relevance to the two questions we have asked. The theory postulated a peripheral origin of migraines ("an irritation in some distant member or viscera"—Willis), followed by a direct internal propagation of the symptoms (by "sympathy" or "consensus"), so that—in the words of Tissot—one part could suffer for another.

Discussion of the basis and mechanisms of migraine still lie far ahead of us, and we raise the specter of "sympathy" not to explain the initiation of migraine attacks (which is a central process), but in relation to the maintenance of attacks already started, and the profound effects which individual symptoms may have on the total attack. Thus, it has always been known that vomiting may rapidly terminate the *entire* migraine attack. An even more commonplace observation is that a simple analgesic (e.g., aspirin) may serve not only to mitigate a migraine headache, but to disperse the *entire* attack. Conversely, it is common knowledge that aggravating a single symptom (as unpleasant smells may increase nausea) may, in turn, aggravate the *entire* attack.

These elementary observations are astonishing in their implications: for they imply that the entire migraine may be perpetuated by one or another of its own symptoms. In short, that a *migraine can become a response to itself.* Given the initial provocation, the original impetus, one may envisage that the subsequent continuance of many migraines may arise in this fashion from a series of self-perpetuating interval drives—a positive feedback—so that the entire reaction is bound within its own circularity. These terms in which one is compelled to think, when faced with the problem of migraines immensely outlasting their provocative circumstances, and protracted beyond any reasonable adaptive (or emotional) function: migraines as self-perpetuating, as fusing stimulus and response, as being held, so to speak, in a corridor of mutually interacting symptoms.*

The role of such self-perpetuating mechanisms may be of particular significance in migraine in view of the fact that *local* tissue changes may occur and prolong individual symptoms (e.g. the train of changes which Wolff has demonstrated following dilatation of extracranial arteries); the persistence of an individual symptom, in this way, may cause the entire attack to persevere.

We must accept, then, that individual symptoms of a migraine can *drive* each other, or indeed the whole attack. Such driving may well be mediated by central reflex arcs, but could also be understood in terms of purely peripheral mechanisms, on the supposition of direct action ("sympathy") between one viscus and another, or rather—putting the old doctrine in modern terms—between one autonomic plexus and another.

Addendum

When the above was written I surmised that a *positive* feedback was involved, a malignant sort of feedback which could keep a

---

*A familiar example of such a peripheral autonomic interaction is the gastrocolic reflex—emptying of the bowel in response to filling of the stomach. This universal postbreakfast reflex is apparently not mediated by central mechanisms at all, but by a direct signalling from stomach to colon, a "sympathy" between these two parts of the gut.

migraine going in a nonadaptive way, long after its initial provocation (and "relevance") were past. I wondered, at the time, whether the converse might hold also, namely, the possibility of a therapeutic or *negative* feedback, which might bring an attack to a speedy end. This is touched on, again, in the final chapter on therapy.

Conclusions

The type of attack we have considered in this chapter must be viewed as radically different from periodic and paroxysmal migraines. The latter gather force and impend in the nervous system; they are set off when they are "due," frequently by trivial or inoffensive stimuli which simply serve to detonate the attack; they run their fixed courses, and are followed by calm. They must be seen as idiopathic events, related primarily to the periodicities of the nervous system. Circumstantial migraines, in contrast, are only elicited by certain *types* of stimulus, and tend to show a significant relation, in their duration and severity, to the strength of this stimulus: thus they are, in essence, graded responses to graded stimuli. The circumstances evocative of these migraines are not trivial or inoffensive; they represent, at least potentially, major disturbances or disruptions or nervous activity. Thus, circumstantial migraines must be viewed not only as neuronal events, but as *reactions* which have a definite function in relation to their provocative circumstances.

We have seen that there are two forms of stimulus which are particularly prone to evoke migrainous reactions in predisposed individuals: inordinate excitations or arousals, and inordinate inhibitions or slumps. Within certain "allowable" limits (which vary greatly from person to person), the nervous system maintains itself in a region of equilibrium, homeostatically, by means of continuous, minor, insensible adjustments; beyond these limits, it may be forced to react to sudden, major, symptomatic adjustments.

Thus, excessive arousal (in the form of sensory bombardment, violent exercise, rage, etc.) tends to be followed by a reaction of prolonged recoil—an arousal migraine; conversely, excessive inhibition (in the form of exhaustion, response to passive motion, etc.) tends to lead, beyond a critical point, to a protracted slump reaction—a slump migraine. In both cases we must envisage a protective function as being carried out by the migraine reaction, a warning to avoid particular circumstances which cannot be tolerated—excessive noise and light, exhaustion, oversleeping, overeating, passive motion, and other occurrences.

Beyond a certain point, we have noted, the migraine may achieve a momentum of its own, and be protracted far beyond what would seem to be any reasonable adaptive function. In such cases, we have postulated, the migraine may be perpetuated as a paradoxical response to itself, a physiological vicious circle.

We have had to consider one type of circumstantial migraine which cannot be fitted into either of the above categories, notably the attacks of aura or classical migraine which may be elicited by flickering light or visualization of a scotoma. We have been compelled to postulate that innate resonance mechanisms form the substrate of such migraines, as is also the case with photogenic epilepsy or photomyoclonus.

Finally, we have had to postulate that migraine, in its capacity as a reaction, is readily amenable to conditioning, and that it may thus become secondarily linked to an enormous variety of idiosyncratic circumstances in the life history of the individual. Only in this way can we explain the bizarre linkings of circumstance and response which seem to defy any possible physiological sense. The final lengths to which such conditioning may go can lead to a singular situation, in which the occurrence of migraine will be linked to the patient's expectation of its occurrence (a familiar analogy to this is seen in the precipitation of an allergic response, an attack of "rose fever," if the patient is shown a paper rose). If this occurs, the patient may become trapped in a circularity of expectations and symptoms, caught in a sort of complicity with himself. A consequence of this, and of the relation between suggestible patients and speculative physicians, is that virtually any theory of migraine may come to generate the data on which it is based.* Cause and effect can become inextricably tangled: as Gibbon has observed, in another connection, "the prediction, as is usual, contributed to its own accomplishment."

---

*The history of hysteria provides many familiar examples of such a merging between expectations and symptoms. Thus Charcot's depiction of hysteria was responsible for the frequent occurrence of the symptoms he depicted. With his death, and the changing of medical expectations, the forms of hysteria changed in turn.

9

Situational Migraine

*There are apparently two essentially different causes [of illness], an inner
one,* causa interna, *which the man contributes of himself, and an outer one,*
causa externa, *which springs from his environment. And accepting this
clear distinction, we have thrown ourselves with raging force upon the
external causes,. . . And the* causa interna, *that we have forgotten. Why?
Because it is not pleasant to look within ourselves. . . .*

—Groddeck

As one receives the history from a migraine patient, the pattern of
his attacks is gradually clarified. It may be obvious, within minutes
of first seeing the patient, that he suffers periodic migraines which
display an innate rhythmicity irrespective of his mode of life, or that
he has attacks which are clearly coupled with one or more of the
provocative circumstances considered in the last chapter. But there
will remain a third group of patients—a large group—who suffer
from repeated and unremitting attacks for no reason which is immediately apparent. Such patients, habitual migraineurs, may have
experienced as many as five attacks weekly for many years, and
they are, therefore, the most cruelly incapacitated of all migraine
sufferers.

Faced with this afflicted group, one must infer that there exists
some chronic situation which "drives" their attacks, some goad
which may be physiological or psychological, intrinsic or extrinsic.
A small minority of these patients seem to suffer from an intrinsic
physiological stimulus to migraine. We may recognize in this category those patients who have had extremely frequent classical migraines or migraine auras from earliest childhood, and who not

uncommonly come from a family background heavily weighted with classical migraine. These rare patients (I have not seen more than half a dozen in my entire experience) appear to have some innate cerebral instability or irritability analogous to severe idiopathic epilepsy. Patients with incessant attacks of migrainous neuralgia, not broken into clusters as is usually the case, may also be the victims of some innate physiological mechanism, and in these one may conceive of some ticlike mechanism, of more peripheral location, analogous to that of trigeminal neuralgia. In a few patients one may discover the importance of certain extrinsic physiological stimuli (e.g., reserpine or hormone medication, the habitual use of alcohol or amphetamines, a particular sensitivity to environmental temperature or illumination, etc.), and be able to exclude these with happy results.

These possibilities will be considered and given a fair hearing by the physician, but by degrees it will be borne in upon him that the vast majority of patients with incessant unremitting migraines are not the victims of such physiological stimuli or sensitivities, but are caught in a malignant emotional "bind" of one sort or another, and *this*, he will come to suspect, is the driving force behind their migraines. Sometimes the emotional stresses, reactions, conflicts, and the like are exposed and plainly in view, so that their existence and possible relevance to the migraine may be evident to both patient and physician. In other patients, the emotional substrates will be hidden and buried, so that their exposure (if this is deemed therapeutic) will be time-consuming and painful, challenging to the utmost the insight and the emotional resources of both patient and physician.

A proportion of patients (perhaps an especially high proportion among sufferers from habitual migraine) and a number of physicians doubt or deny that migraine can be a psychosomatic illness, and commit themselves to an endless search for physiological causes and pharmacological treatments. Physicians who are prepared to think in terms of psychosomatic mechanisms have studied their patients in either of two ways. The first method of study is to investigate the features of the patient's personality and life situation as far as these are accessible in ordinary medical practice; such methods, necessarily, provide a relatively superficial picture of the patient's problems, but have the advantage that great numbers of patients may be submitted to observation (a classic among such studies was Wolff's investigation of forty-six migraine patients).

The second method of study is a psychoanalytic one, and possible only in the very protracted and special conditions of an analysis; here the patient is studied in immense depth, but such investigations have the disadvantage that only a handful of patients are submitted to observation (a classic among such psychoanalytic studies is that of Fromm-Reichmann).

These two groups of investigators tend to use different languages, and their conclusions may therefore be difficult to compare. Furthermore, they are concerned with different aspects of the patient's emotional being, the first group being concerned with the overall features of overt personality, and the analysts with unconscious and often deeply hidden emotional transactions in the psyche. There has been, nevertheless, a considerable unanimity of opinion with regard to the types of patient, and types of emotional posture, that may be seen in relation to habitual migraine. Wolff (1963) has delineated the features of the "migraine personality" in greater detail than all his predecessors. Migraineurs are portrayed by Wolff as ambitious, successful, perfectionistic, rigid, orderly, cautious, and emotionally constipated, driven therefore, from time to time, to outbursts and breakdowns which must assume an indirect, somatic form. Fromm-Reichmann (1937) is also able to arrive at a clear-cut conclusion: migraine, she states, is a physical expression of unconscious hostility against consciously beloved persons.

My own method of study has been more akin to Wolff's and has allowed me to interview many hundreds of migraine patients. In a number of cases (including those presented in this chapter) I have been able to see patients twice a month for prolonged periods, and thus gain some insight into problems which would not have been apparent on a single interview, or even half a dozen interviews. I have not had the opportunity, and I have lacked the skills, for protracted depth-analysis of my patients.

During the early days of practice with migraine patients, and fresh from the literature on the subject, I tried to recognize, in every patient with habitual migraine that I saw, Wolff's stereotype of the "migraine personality," or Fromm-Reichmann's subtler qualities of ambivalence and repressed hostility. I was forced to the conclusion, by degrees, that neither of these generalizations had

e to more than a proportion of the patients I saw. On the
y, patients with severe habitual migraine seemed to me
ious in their emotional pathologies and predicaments that I
aired of putting them in a single category, unless I played
crustes.

There is persuasive evidence that chronic emotional need of a
particular type characterize, for example, the majority of patients
with peptic ulcers (see Alexander and French, 1948), but the analogy
between such a psychosomatic disorder and habitual migraine is
difficult to maintain. It appears, on the contrary, that migraines may
be summoned to serve an endless variety of emotional ends. As
migraines may assume a remarkable diversity of forms, so they may
carry as various a load of emotional implications. If they are the
most common of psychosomatic reactions, it is because they are the
most versatile.

Case Histories

Case 76

This 43-year-old woman, a nun, had been subject to frequent common
migraines and stuporous migraine equivalents since the age of 17, when
she entered the religious life. Eleven months of each year were spent in
the convent, and during these eleven months the patient would suffer two
or three attacks of migraine, or migraine equivalent, weekly. She received
one month of holiday annually, and during this she would rarely have even
one attack.

Comment: This patient was an energetic, well-integrated if somewhat impatient person, a woman of strong practical ability who
enjoyed exercise and fresh air, conversation and the theater. Her
strong sense of duty and altruism had been a main factor in directing
her into religious life. The claustrophobic conditions of convent life,
the dearth of opportunities for physical and social activity, and
above all the restriction of frank emotional expression appeared to
be the main factors in driving this patient to somatic expression.
Irritability, anger, sulking, and other such behavior were not permissible in the convent, but migraine was. Given freedom from
restrictions and impediments she immediately lost the need for her
attacks.

Case 78

This case was a 55-year-old woman with thrice-weekly attacks of common migraine. When questioned about her personal life, she admitted to constant anxiety concerning her husband, a diabetic prone to frequent and frightening insulin-reactions.

Her husband, a depressive with strong sadomasochistic traits, confessed, when interviewed alone, that he "guessed" how much insulin to take, and felt it "unnecessary" to test his urine for sugar. He was persuaded, with some difficulty, to place himself under competent medical care, and forthwith ceased to experience further insulin-reactions. With their disappearance, his wife became virtually exempt from migraine, and in a six-month follow-up had suffered only two attacks.

Comment: This patient had been living in a chronic anxiety state, almost wholly bound up with her husband's illness. It might also be speculated that she wished to "join him" in a pattern of recurrent illness. With his liberation from illness her level of anxiety at once declined, and her migraines turned from habitual to occasional.

Case 79

A 46-year-old woman with three highly intelligent, demanding, "difficult" and excessively loved adolescent children. This patient had experienced very occasional migraines prior to the adolescence of her children, but had been subject to two or more attacks weekly since their entering their stormy puberties. Expressions of affection and maternal solicitude alternated with outbreaks of irritability. Each summer the loved but difficult children were dispatched to youth camps, and for three months the patient would be relieved of her anxieties, her irritability, and her migraine.

Comment: This situation, a common one in many parents, especially mothers, whom I have seen, is perhaps the best example of Fromm-Reichmann's theory.

Case 80

A 42-year-old woman with exceedingly frequent, and at times "almost continuous" migraine attacks, who complained that half of her waking hours were spent suffering, and a third of them in bed.

When questioned about her personal life, she smiled and maintained that everything was "beautiful," her husband "a perfect gentleman," and her children "lovely." She vehemently denied that there were any problems of any sort. "There is not a cloud in the sky," she would say; "I have nothing to complain of except this wretched migraine."

Over the course of several months, in which other members of the family were seen, it became apparent that there were innumerable problems. The family was in debt and heavily mortgaged, the husband was impotent, and the eldest child was a drop-out from school and a juvenile delinquent.

Comment: Here we see a situation with some similarities to the last case, but altogether more serious and pathological. The patient displays a hysterical denial and repression of all "bad" emotional feelings, and maintains a set of conscious attitudes wholly at variance with the realities of her position. She is, indeed, "split" into two selves: one portion of her consists of denial and bravado, the other a split-off system inflicting illness upon itself, and suffering continually.

Case 81

This 55-year-old man had been a former inmate of Auschwitz. He had suffered about one attack of classic migraine a month from the age of 7 until his incarceration in Auschwitz. During his six years in the concentration camp—six years during which his wife, parents, and all other close relatives were killed—he did not experience a single attack of migraine. He was liberated by the Allies in 1945, and the following year emigrated to the United States.

Since this time, he has been chronically depressed, guilt-ridden, preoccupied with the deaths of all his relatives whom he feels he might have saved, and intermittently psychotic. During this time he has also experienced six to ten attacks of classical migraine each month, attacks which are refractory to treatment, and accompanied by the most intense suffering.

He is also considerably accident-prone, and during the two years that I saw him he managed to sustain a Colles fracture, a fracture dislocation of one ankle, and a head injury. Each of these injuries was followed by several weeks' remission of his migraines. It is also of interest that on the three occasions in which he has been hospitalized for psychotic depressions during the past twenty years, he was free from migraines.

Comment: This tragic case history illustrates several points of interest. The exemption from migraine during his years in a concentration camp is a feature which has been described to me by several other patients: all forms of psychosomatic illness, and also frank psychosis, were apparently extremely rare in such conditions, presumably because they would have been lethally maladaptive. Since this time he has been frankly and greatly depressed, and has fully conscious, constantly reiterated, feelings of self-accusation and wishes for self-punishment.

His migraines gratify and reinforce such feelings, being sadistically inflicted and masochistically suffered. Sometimes an "accident" will serve a similar function, and thus dispense for a while with the necessity of migraines. When his depression reaches psychotic intensity and he feels himself to be in the hell he deserves, his hallucinations and delusions similarly dispense with the relatively inconsiderable migraines.

Case 56

A 43-year-old woman who had suffered severe common migraines, usually two or three attacks a month, since childhood. She could recollect only three periods during which she had been exempt from attacks: during a severe illness (subacute bacterial endocarditis), when she was in hospital for four months; during her first three pregnancies, when she went more than six months without attacks (this was in dramatic contrast to her fourth, unwanted, pregnancy, when she not only continued to have migraines throughout the nine months, but had more severe attacks than usual for her); finally, during a three-month period when she was mourning for her father to whom she had been deeply attached.

Comment: That is, as it were, a case history in reverse, showing certain situations in which a patient found herself *free* from life-long migraines, and as such supplements the preceding case history. Exemption from migraine during pregnancy is a very common experience, and has generally been ascribed to the physiological or hormonal changes occurring during pregnancy (see chapters 8 and 10). The above case history suggests that psychological factors must also be taken into account: the four pregnancies were, one may presume, physiologically similar, but the last of them was unique in being undesired by the patient. Freedom from migraine (and many other psychosomatic symptoms) is often procured during severe illnesses, and one must wonder whether medical attention, social support and sympathy, in conjunction with release from many habitual stresses, are perhaps the "liberating" factors, rather than the illness *per se*. Mourning, in which the free expression of emotion receives social support and sympathy, may absolve a patient from migraine and similar symptoms, in distinction to depressive reactions which tend to aggravate these.

Case 82

A 40-year-old woman who, when first seen, was suffering from a severe migraine and accompanied by her husband who took it upon himself to provide the "history." This he did with sadistic relish, disguised as "scientific detachment." A statistician, he had gone to extraordinary lengths to note the dates of every attack his wife had experienced in the past four years, compared these with the dates of her menstrual periods, the vagaries of her diet, changes in the weather, and the like. He had computed correlation coefficients for all these "factors." Much of his time was evidently spent ministering to his wife, for he served as her physician, and computed with equal care precisely what drugs she should receive in each attack. Both he and she emphasize the necessity of frequent ergotamine and pethidine (Demerol) injections.

Comment: This case history is essentially one of a *folie à deux* between two people who are both symbiotically and destructively dependent upon each other. The sexual aspects of their marriage had long since foundered, but had been replaced, apparently, by a sadomasochistic intimacy revolving around the patient's migraines.

Case 84

This patient, a 44-year-old man, had been employed for many years by an uncle whom he loathed. The conditions of work were unpleasant, and were made worse by his employer's habitual sarcasms; the salary, however, was considerably in excess of what the patient might have earned in comparable work elsewhere, and this had made him reluctant to seek "outside" employment. He suffered from continual belching and frequent migraines, two or three attacks weekly, throughout his working year, but was free of these during his annual monthly vacation.

Comment: This patient was caught in a dilemma in which humiliating conditions of work had been "accepted" for financial reward. Caught in a situation of deeply resented bondage, he felt himself unable to improve his working conditions, or seek employment elsewhere. Ostensibly mute and compliant, he expressed his rage in physiological terms, as continued eructations and migraines.

Case 55

This 42-year-old man had once aspired to the priesthood, but was frustrated in this ambition. He lived a querulous and joyless existence, masochistically bound to his domineering mother with whom he lived. Seven or eight times a year, desire would override guilt, and he would steal out of the house to seek sexual contact. Within five minutes of orgasm a "terrible" migraine would come upon him, and rack him with pain for the ensuing three days.

Comment: This guilt-ridden Catholic had morbid fears of sexual intercourse, which he construed as a sin richly deserving of punishment. His migraines provided the requisite punishment, three days of cephalgic penance, after which he regained his physiological and moral equilibrium.

Case 62

A 55-year-old woman whose symptoms were briefly described in chapter 2. Unmarried, and the only daughter of parents who had always been demanding and possessive, and were now ageing and in poor health, she was compelled to work at two jobs, for a total of fourteen hours daily, to support the household. She had no friends, no social life, and had never had any sexual experience. She felt it her "duty" to support her parents and to be with them whenever she was not working.

At one time, indeed, she had made pathetic efforts to establish an independent existence, but these had been foiled first by parental intervention, and subsequently by her own discomfort and guilt if she went out alone. In the past ten years she had lost all choice in the matter, for she suffered severely from migraine, ulcerative colitis, and psoriasis, not concurrently, but in a never-ending cycle.

Comment: This pitiful case history illustrates the sacrifice of a life, and the trapping of this patient at three concentric levels: an intolerable domestic reality, an intolerable neurotic conflict, and an intolerable circle of psychosomatic symptoms.

Case 83

A 35-year-old engineer, this patient had founded, and directed, a highly successful "thought tank," a group which offered computing and mathematical research work for many industrial and governmental concerns. Brilliant and insatiably ambitious, this patient drove himself and his subordinates to ruthless extremes.

He worked incessantly every evening and all Saturday. He permitted himself no hobbies, no social life, and no children. Every Sunday morning he would wake with a severe migraine. Originally he had forced himself to work despite the headache, but for the past two years the attacks had been accompanied by such nausea and vomiting that he was incapacitated for the day.

Comment: Here we see a patient with such a hypertrophied "drive" that he would work a seven-day week, or even a 168-hour week, if it were humanly possible. But it is not humanly possible, and his human limits were enforced by regular Sunday migraines which acted as physiological Sabbaths. This patient is the only one in the above series who has a "migraine personality."

Conclusions

We have concluded that the majority of patients who experience very frequent, severe, and unremitting migraines, for which no obvious circumstantial antecedents can be traced, are reacting to chronically difficult, intolerable, and even frightful life situations. In such patients we are able to observe or to infer powerful emotional stresses and needs, and to realize that these are driving recurrent attacks. Of this species of migraine, and no other, we may legitimately use the term "psychosomatic illness." Such illnesses represent (in Borges' magnificent phrase) "apparent desperations and secret assuagements." We have noted, in one case history, the alternation of migraines with another form of somatic assuagement— repeated accidents—and we might have presented much evidence regarding the alternation or replacement of migraines with repeated minor viral illnesses (colds, upper respiratory infections, herpes, etc.) and allergic manifestations, which may also, apparently, be pressed into similar roles in the emotional economy.

We believe that migraine may be adopted as an expression of emotional stress and distress of many different types, and that it is impossible to fit all patients into the stereotype of the obsessive "migraine personality," or to find in all of them chronic repressed rage and hostility. Nor should one claim that all patients with habitual migraine are "neurotic" (except in so far as neurosis is the universal human condition), for in many cases—a matter which will receive full discussion in Part III—the migraines may replace a neurotic structure, constituting an alternative to neurotic desperation and assuagement.

Part III

The BASIS
of MIGRAINE

10

Physiological Changes in Migraine Attacks

The migraine sufferer knows directly what he experiences—*he* is the authority on his own experience. He does not know what goes on beneath the level of experience, in the different nerve cells, tissues, and systems of his brain. A knowledge of the underlying physiology of migraine is necessary for the physician who is to treat it scientifically, and vital for the development of new drugs and therapies: it was discussed in detail in the original edition, because this was *aimed* at physicians, and teachers, and researchers, no less than it was aimed at the patient himself. This new edition, by contrast, is aimed almost solely at the patient—and the public—and can therefore dispense with the elaborate detail and discussion of the original.

Here, then, we aim at a summary outline—a brief guide to the underlying physiology of migraine, which the patient can relate to his own experiences, and to whatever therapeutic measures seem appropriate for him.

When Liveing came to consider the physiology of migraine, a little over a century ago, he discussed it under the following main heads:

(1) *Vasomotor theories*—which tried to relate the symptoms of migraine to changes in blood vessels in the brain and the head.
(2) *Humoral theories*—or, as we would now call them, chemical theories.
(3) *Electrical theories*—and his own theory of "nerve-storms."

We can hardly do better, a century later, than follow this very general classification; it can at least form a framework and springboard for discussion.

There is no vasomotor theory of migraine which had not been considered a century ago. It was considered then that there was a double effect: first a *contraction* of the cranial vessels, due to excessive vasomotor tone; and then an *expansion* and loss of vessel tone. It was widely felt that this expansion and dilatation of vessels—branches of the carotid artery in the temples and scalp—was the cause of migraine headache (when it occurred). On the other hand, there was considerable doubt as to whether contraction of cerebral vessels could cause the much more complex features of the aura. Gowers, in particular, was very critical of this notion, and wrote:

That vasomotor spasm can cause a deliberate, uniform, and peculiar "discharge" is not only unproved, but in the highest degree improbable.

It is now possible to demonstrate—by such techniques as thermography, and measuring cerebral blood flow—that there is, indeed, such a vasomotor action; and it is possible to prove that the headache itself is a consequence of dilatation in certain extracranial arteries (usually the superficial temporal artery, which may be felt in each temple), followed by the exudation of pain-producing fluid. If we prevent this dilatation of extracranial arteries, we can prevent the vascular headache of migraine—but cause very little change to the *other* features of migraine—its aura, its visceral effects, its irritability, and other phenomena.

What Gowers wrote a century ago remains true today—that vasomotor changes usefully explain the cause of migraine *headache*, but do nothing to explain the origin of migraine *attacks* (the whole complex attack of which the headache is a small and secondary part).

If we wish for an understanding of migraine *attacks*, we must turn away from vasomotor changes, and consider chemical and electrical changes in the brain.

We have observed from the start that migraine attacks involve changes in the *tonus* of the nervous system, especially those parts which we call "vegetative" or "autonomic." The tone, or tuning of the nervous system, and, in particular, its autonomic parts, is mediated by various *neurotransmitters*, which are involved in the transmission of nerve impulses from one nerve cell to another.

There are upwards of a dozen neurotransmitters in the nervous system. Each of these perform specific transmitter-functions, but none of them acts in isolation from the rest. Measurements have been made of most of the neurotransmitters in migraine—and we find ourselves with a *surfeit* of chemical information! There is evidence that *all* natural neurotransmitters may show significant changes during an attack of migraine—and often in its premonitory stages as well.

We see changes in adrenalin, nor-adrenalin, acetylcholine, histamine; and, often prominently, in 5-hydroxy-tryptamine (or serotonin).

Certain evidence with regard to the experimental induction of attacks, and their therapeutic termination, indicates that serotonin may often play a role. But one must stress the word *often*, and distinguish it from "always"; there may be several different sorts of migraine, which are *chemically* distinct, and the specific therapy for each would be different. Again the persistence of migraines, following experimental *block* of this transmitter or that, suggest there may be a choice in chemical terms—and that if an attack is going to occur, it *will* occur, irrespective of what is blocked.

This compulsive, and indeed convulsive, quality of migraines is very marked—especially in regard to classical migraine and migraine aura. If migraine is indeed a "nerve-storm," a sort of vegetative epilepsy, or epilepsy-in-slow-motion, one would hope to find *electrical evidence* of the sort that is so common, and valuable, in seizures.

Unfortunately, this lead—which might seem the best one we have—runs into unexpected difficulties of all kinds. Electroencephalography (EEG), which allows us to monitor the electrical activity of the brain through the use of recording electrodes on the scalp, requires complex apparatus, and fairly complex setting up. If we could wire up the patient, and then *give* him a migraine—preferably an acute attack, best of all a migraine aura—we might stand a better chance of picking up information. Unfortunately, we have no sure method of inducing a migraine—certainly not a migraine aura; and the chances of "catching" one are not very good. Sometimes, however, luck may prevail, and there have been some impressive recordings in migraine auras, which have shown "spikes" on the EEG, in the visual areas, which are very similar to the spikes one may see in seizures. But this finding is not constant: one may monitor the patient during a severe migraine aura, and *fail* to find any spikes at all.*

That *some* form of electrical disturbance accompanies a migraine can hardly be doubted, but the nature of this disturbance is still quite unclear. It has been estimated by physiologists, themselves prone to scotomata, that scotomatous enlargement corresponds to a wave of excitation (or depression) moving across the visual cortex at about 3 mm per minute (Lashley, 1941). But electrical activity this slow—about a hundred times slower than an epileptic seizure—cannot be monitored by present-day methods.

The Origin of Migraine

The general *picture* of migraine, in physiological terms, can scarcely be better put than it was put by Liveing: a sort of slow seizure, or reaction, starting deep in the brainstem, and which is projected upwards on to the cerebral cortex, and downwards and peripherally to the plexuses of the body—the nerve nets about viscera, blood vessels, glands. We must see the upward projection to the cortex as kindling within it the phenomena of the aura—scotomata, paresthesia, and so on, and the peripheral projections as kindling local excitements in the nerve nets manifest as vascular headache, borborygmi, salivation, and other occurrences.

The Place of Migraine

The notion of "borderlands" is not just a figure of speech, but an indication of physiological affinity and contiguity. Gowers spoke of migraines as located in the borderlands of epilepsy, and we may imagine it, similarly, on the borders of sleep, and sometimes on the borders of delirium and madness. Perhaps we should envisage a cosmography or geography of human nature, with all its possibilities

*Very recently, working with my electroencephalographer, Mrs. P. C. Carolan, I have had the extraordinary luck of monitoring the EEG in two patients—identical twin sisters—during the course of a severe scotomatous ("blind") migraine aura. In both cases we saw enormous slow waves down in the delta range (1-3 Hz) confined to the occipital electrodes, which disappeared in a few minutes as the patients regained their vision.

and phenomena set out in relation—like a map of the heavens, or a map of the world. One such map was attempted in *figure 7*; another is depicted in *figure 8* below, inscribing migraine, and bordering disorders, in terms of time base and neural level.

Migraine and neighboring disorders are here represented in terms of time base and neural level; either of these may be modulated—hence the metamorphoses to which migraine is prone. All of the disorders here represented are distinct and individual, but nevertheless have borderlands in which they merge into another.

Migraine as a "Task"

It was suggested, as early as the Preface of this book, that migraines had to be seen as both *structures* and *strategies*. We have, roughly, visualized them now as a tactic or "task."

A. R. Luria has done more than anyone else in analyzing the organization of movements and *motor* tasks, and the concepts and terms he uses seem equally applicable to an event like a migraine which may constitute a *vegetative* task or action.

According to the thinking of Luria and his school, a *function* is in fact a *functional system* directed toward the performance of a par-

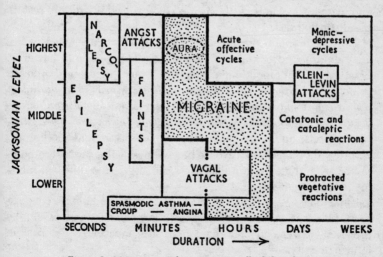

Figure 8. Migraine in relation to some allied disorders

ticular biological task. The most significant feature of such a functional system is that it is based on a dynamic "constellation" of connections, situated at different levels in the nervous system, and that *these* may be freely substituted for one another or interchanged with the task itself remaining unchanged. Thus (in Luria's words) "such a system of functionally united components has a systematic, not a concrete, structure, in which the initial and final links of the system (the task and the effect) remain constant and unchanged, while the intermediate links (the means of performance of the task) may be modified within wide limits."

These considerations, discussed by Luria in reference to movement and motor tasks, recommend themselves as indispensable for the understanding of migraine and its transformations as *autonomic and psychosomatic tasks*. The task may be shaped by the necessity of neuronal discharge (in a periodic or paroxysmal migraine), or by physical or emotional need(s), as in circumstantial or situational attacks; the final link, the effects of the migraine, is the restoration of a physiological (or emotional) equilibrium. But the adaptive task has a systematic and not a concrete structure, that is, *the actual mechanisms employed may be many, various, and inconstant*. There may be as many ways of concocting a migraine as of cooking an omelette. If one particular intermediate link, one mechanism, is eliminated, the whole system can be reorganized in order to restore the disturbed task.

Thus, as in motor or perceptual tasks, the particular mechanisms are subordinated to the overall strategy. This principle has great practical and therapeutic importance as well as theoretical interest. It means, for example, that *if migraine is necessary in the physiological or emotional economy of an individual, attacks will continue to occur, to be elaborated, whatever particular mechanisms are eliminated*. Excise one temporal artery, one end-organ, and another will be pressed into use; endeavor to block attacks with, say, a serotonin-inhibitor, and attacks are likely to recur utilizing a different intermediate mechanism.

Functional systems such as these (says Luria), complex in composition, *plastic in the variability of their elements*, and possessing the property of dynamic autoregulation, are apparently the rule in human activity.

11

Biological Approaches
to Migraine

We would hesitate to recognize in animals anything which might be termed a *migraine*, and this, among other factors, has limited the experimental investigation of the subject. Must we then regard migraines as peculiar to our own species? Speech is predominant in man, and certain very sophisticated reactions (Darwin instances laughing, frowning and sneering) are exclusively found in man, but these activities and reactions are not usefully compared to migraines. Migraine, in contrast to these, is a remarkably primitive reaction involving massive alternations of vegetative activity and of general activity and behavior. We have considered migraine, thus far, in chiefly experiential terms, as the symptoms of which a patient may complain, and at this level, obviously, we can derive no information from animals which may suffer but cannot express complaints. If we are to form any picture of the biological role(s) of migraine, and of its corresponding analogies in the animal world, we must instead concern ourselves with the *behavior* of the migraine patient, and the circumstances to which this behavior has relevance.

Let us then construct a stereotyped picture of migrainous behavior. As the symptoms mount, the patient will go to his room and lie down; he will have the blinds drawn and the children hushed; he will tolerate no intrusions. The intensity of his symptoms will drive other thoughts from his mind; he may be sunk if the attack is very severe, in a leaden, stuporous daze. He pulls the blanket over his head, excluding the outer world, and enveloping himself in the inner world of his symptoms. He says to the world: "Go away. Leave me alone. This is my migraine. Let me suffer in peace." At length, perhaps, he falls asleep. And when he wakes, it is all over, the migraine is done, its work is accomplished; there may be a postmigrainous surge of energy, almost literally a reanimation. The essential terms of the attack are these: retreat from the outer world, regression, and, finally, recuperation.

In somewhat less formal terms, the migraine reaction tends to be characterized by passivity, stillness and immobilization; commerce with the outer world in minimal, while inner activities—particularly of secretory and expulsive type—are maximal. It is in *these* general terms that we may perceive the primary adaptive function of a migraine (whatever complex uses are subsequently superimposed), and in these terms that we may seek for parallel reactions both in the human and the animal world.

It is particularly as a protective reflex that we envisage the primary role of migraine, as a withdrawal of the whole body from "the operation of a noxious or endangering stimulus," in short, as a *particular form of reaction to threat*.

Response to threat, in the animal world, may take either or both of two fundamentally different forms. The form which is most familiar, and which springs immediately to mind, is the use of an active physical response, the fight-flight response, with its emotional correlates of rage or terror. The general mechanisms of this have been incomparably described by Cannon (1920) with respect to acute reactions, and by Selye (1946) in regard to sustained physiological reactions. The acute fight-flight picture is one of extreme arousal and sympathetic dominance: muscles tensed, deepened breathing, increased cardiac output, extreme sensory vigilance, every external faculty keyed to its highest pitch, and a reciprocal inhibition of internal (parasympathetically driven) processes. The acute reaction induces and is reinforced by the secretion of adrenalin and other pressor amines, while the chronic reaction involves adrenocortical activity and a chain of chemical and tissue reactions secondary to this.

The fight-flight reaction is dramatic in the extreme, but it represents only half of biological reality. The other half is no less dramatic, but it is dramatic in a contrary style. *Its* characteristics are those of passivity and immobilization in response to threat. The antithesis between these two styles of reaction was memorably described by Darwin in his comparison of active fear (terror) and passive fear (dread). In the former, says Darwin, there is "the sudden and uncontrollable tendency to headlong flight." The picture of passive fear, as Darwin portrays it, is one of passivity and prostration, allied with increased splanchnic and glandular activity ("a strong tendency to yawn . . . death-like pallor . . . beads of sweat stand out on the skin. All of the muscles of the body are relaxed. Utter prostration soon follows. The intestines are affected. The sphincter muscles cease to act, and no longer retain the contents of the body . . . "). The general attitude is one of cringing, cowering, and sinking. If the passive reaction is more acute, there may be abrupt loss of postural tone or of consciousness. If the passive reaction is more protracted, the physiological changes are less dramatic, but still in the same direction.

We find throughout the animal world a repertoire of passive reactions at least as important as and considerably more variable than the active responses to threat. All of them are characterized by immobilization (with some inhibition of postural tone and arousal), usually in conjunction with increased secretory and splanchnic activity. A handful of examples will suffice. A fearful dog cowers, and may vomit and be incontinent of feces; the hedgehog responds to threat by curling up; the gerbil by a sudden cataplectic loss of muscular tone; the opossum by a trancelike arrest or "sham death." The frightened horse may "freeze" and break into a cold sweat; the threatened skunk freezes and secretes profusely from modified sweat glands (here the secretory response has assumed an offensive function); the menaced chameleon freezes and changes color to mimic the environment through another variant of internal secretion. Even in the protozoa, we find active, predatory responses in some groups, and passive protective responses in others. It is clear that the passive response to threat has been utilized, from the start of life, as a biological alternative to active reactions. The passive reaction, indeed, is frequently superior to the active response in terms of survival value. Where the aroused animal faces (or flees) danger and threat, the inhibitory reaction enables it to *avert* these, to become, one way or another, less accessible to danger.

The human repertoire is particularly rich in such passive protective reactions many of which occur paradoxically in the context of physical or emotional crisis. Among such relatively acute reactions we must rank narcolepsy and cataplexy, nervous "freezing" and

"blocking," an enormous variety of Parkinsonian "crises,"* and fainting. On a somewhat more extended time scale we see vasovagal
attacks and, of course, migraines. We must also recognize as inhibitory protective reactions such states as "swooning" (hysterical
stupor), and much more protracted depressive and catatonic
stupors. Pathological sleeping (especially in its most baroque form
of trance or catalepsy) is the exemplar of the longer-lasting human
inhibitory reactions, as is hibernation in the animal world.

The survival-value of passive reactions and inhibitory states is
clearly apparent in the animal world, whereas it tends to be
obscured or overshadowed in some of the more obviously pathological passive reactions in human behavior. But we will find it
impossible to comprehend the origin and perpetuation of such
human reactions unless they are seen, first and foremost, as having
biological survival value. Paradox is implicit in the nature of such
reactions; sleep and hibernation serve to protect the organism, but
may also expose it to other vicissitudes. Inhibitory, parasympathetically dominated states in man may afford a "vegetative retreat," but
the seclusion of retreat may become a psychophysiological imprison-
ment. The ultimate paradox is the simulation of death to avoid
death, as we see in the "sham death" of the opossum and, perhaps,
some human sleeps and stupors.

This then is the hinterland of biological reactions from which we
conceive migraines to have arisen in the course of evolution,
and to have become, with the elaboration of human nervous
systems and human needs, progressively differentiated and refined.
Our image is of a primal migraine, or archetype, a crude passive-
protective-parasympathetic type of reaction of longer duration than
the common freezing and stun reactions. Perhaps such primordial
migraines—similar to the undifferentiated reactions considered in
chapter 2—were chiefly in response to a variety of physical threats:
exhaustion, heat, illness, injury, pain, and the like, and certain
elemental and overwhelming emotional experiences, especially fear.

The development of large social units, and the cultural repressions
inseparable from this, have doubtless necessitated, as they have
permitted, a far greater variety of vegetative retreats and protracted
passive reactions than were previously possible. These psychosoma-

*Described in *Awakenings*.

tic reactions, along with neurotic defenses and reactions, represent the only alternatives in situations where direct action is neither permissible nor possible. We envisage that psychosomatic reactions, like neurotic defences, have become not only more necessary with the increasing complexity and repressiveness of civilized life, but also more versatile and sophisticated: thus, the simple protective reflexes we have discussed may evolve into the richly allusive, overdetermined, and variable migraines so common in present society.

Proceeding parallel with the elaboration of such strategic needs and uses has been the increasing complexity of the nervous system, and in particular, the progressive encephalization of integrative functions in the course of mammalian evolution. In relatively primitive mammals (opossums, hedgehogs, etc.) in which cortical development and control are rudimentary, cerebral reflexes must still be of relatively stereotyped form and little susceptible of conditioning. The elaboration of the cortical mantle permits the unfolding of more numerous, more various, and more easily conditioned cerebral reflexes.

Thus to the question posed at the start of this chapter—is migraine a uniquely human reaction?—we must answer yes and no. It makes no sense to regard migraine as a human invention. We must see it, rather, as having a most ancient lineage of biological precursors, as exemplifying a most primitive and generalized form of adaptive reaction which has been refined and differentiated by the unique possibilities of human nervous systems and the unique nature of human needs.

12

Psychological Approaches to Migraine

Socrates, in Plato, would prescribe no Physick for Charmides' headache till first he had eased his troublesome mind; body and soul must be cured together, as head and eyes . . .

—Burton

We were concerned in the last chapter with certain primitive reactions which might throw some clue on the origin and differentiation of the human migraine reaction. We take it as axiomatic that every attack of migraine has tactical value to the person (the tactic may be a purely physiological one, e.g., a homeostatic maneuver), but we will be particularly concerned, in the present chapter, with the relation of migraines to the patient's emotional being.

We made a somewhat arbitrary classification of migraines in the descriptive portion of this book, and we must now examine this classification more closely in so far as it may be related to the emotional economy of an individual. "Periodic" migraines were portrayed as the expression of some innate neuronal periodicity, and "circumstantial" migraines as a response to highly specific, individual circumstances which might be physiological (exhaustion, etc.) or emotional (rage, fright, etc.). The fact that such attacks may have clearly defined physical or physiological antecedents does not exclude the possibility that they may *also* have other functions or uses which may not be immediately apparent. In particular, any attack of migraine (and indeed any event in a person's existence) may be invested with an emotional significance over and above its literal significance. A periodically recurring or physiologically induced event may be pressed into service as a symbolic event.

It is not suggested that all people and circumstantial migraines, or even a majority of them, are coupled in this manner to the motives of the individual. Many migraines occur, pass, constitute occasional inconveniences, and carry no special load of emotional implication. But the possibility of their serving other purposes, of many and various kinds, is always present.

The third pattern of migraines described—habitual or situational migraine—demands a much more complex frame of reference. We are here concerned, not with periodic or sporadic attacks that may or may not have some emotional significance, but with an unremitting, malignant illness, which is generated by (and itself may aggravate) chronic, severe, emotional stresses. The origins and primordia of migraine may be discerned, we have imagined, among simple protective reflexes and tactics. Circumstantial migraines may also be discussed in such terms, given the special reservations we have made. Habitual migraine cannot be usefully considered save as an expression of a major portion of the entire personality. Habitual migraine, like all psychosomatic illnesses, like hysteria, like neurosis, is among the most complex of human creations.

We have already indicated by a number of case histories some of the motives that may generate habitual migraines (chapter 9), and we will now venture to tabulate the major strategic roles that migraines may play in the economy of the individual. The list is incomplete and schematic, of necessity, and cannot do justice to the complexity and flux of the forces that are actually at work, and that tend to interact and combine with one another, so that many migraine attacks are as richly overdetermined as dreams.

Biologically the simplest, and dynamically the most benign of migraines, are *recuperative*. These tend to occur, circumstantially, following prolonged physical or emotional activity, and habitually as the notorious "weekend" attacks. There is usually a rather sharp collapse from the preceding or provocative period of overactivity and tension, the phase of prostration may be profound and even stuporous, and it is followed, characteristically, by a postmigrainous rebound and sense of awakening and reanimation. Wolff has particularly concerned himself with attacks of this type, and their occurrence as "let-down" phenomena in ruthlessly obsessive and driving personalities. Recuperative attacks have the closest biological analogy to sleep, and are clearly preservative reflexes.

Allied to these, geared to environmental or emotional stress, but less benign in their pattern, are those migraines that are *regressive*. Like recuperative migraines, these afford (in Alexander's phrase) a "vegetative retreat"; but whereas recuperative attacks tend to be undertaken in privacy and solitude, like sleep, regressive attacks are marked by pitiful suffering, dependency needs, and cries for help. In a word, they assume the characteristics not of sleep, but of illness. Severe ones, in family contexts, may radiate the tragic qualities of death-bed scenes. Regressive migraines are not infrequently found in the context of illness-prone or hypochondriacal personalities, and are often presented, to the physician, in the context of multiple physical complaints, real or imaginary. We have observed that their pattern may be less benign than that of recuperative migraines: we are here considering not the occasional regressive attacks which any migraineur may have, but an indulgence, a morbid welcoming, of such attacks with ever-increasing frequency, so that the patient slips, by degrees, into illness as a way of life ("that long disease, my life").

An extremely important variant of such migraine patterns, and one which continues to show the primal protective role of the migraine reaction, are those attacks that we may term *encapsulative* and *dissociative*. There are a number of patients in whom periodic or sporadic migraines are experienced which seem to embed, and (in the oblique terms of a physiological drama) to enact and "work through" an accumulation of emotional stresses and conflicts. I have the impression that many menstrual migraines (and other allied menstrual syndromes) do exactly this, condensing, as it were, the stresses of the month into a few days of concentrated illness, and I have observed, in a number of patients, that curing them (depriving them) of such menstrual syndromes may be followed by a release of diffuse anxiety and neurotic conflict into the remainder of the month. Such migraines, in a word, may serve to *bind*, and thus circumscribe, painful chronic or recurrent feelings, a consideration which must be borne in mind before they are too zealously dispersed. More malignant than these, for the emotional substrates are more intense and much farther removed from consciousness, and the migraines, correspondingly, are far more frequent, is that pattern of habitual migraine we have termed dissociative. In such cases (see, for example, case 80) the personality becomes sectioned, one part of it affirming a bland reaction or bravura wholly at odds with environmental and emotional reality, and another portion becoming autonomized as a circular sadomasochistic system devoted to the infliction and experiencing of suffering. Such cases, which are often of the greatest severity, may be peculiarly resistant to insight or treatment, for the migrainous portion of the personality is likely to be insulated from the remainder of the personality by thick walls of repression and denial. The dynamics and mechanisms of this bear the closest analogy to those involved in the formation of hysterical symptoms, with the important difference that migraines are rooted in physiological reactivity, whereas hysterical symptoms (though intensely real) are fictions, neurologically, arising from a pathology of the imagination.

The last two categories of migraine pattern we must consider are distinguished by having acquired special strategic significances of a peculiarly hostile type. The first of these is the *aggressive* migraine, and it is with this type that Fromm-Reichmann (1937), Johnson (1948), and many other analysts have particularly concerned themselves. The emotional background is one of intense, chronic, repressed rage and hostility, and the function of the migraines is to provide some expression of what cannot be expressed, or even acknowledged, directly. Such migraines are implicit assaults or vengeful attacks, and tend to occur in situations of intense emotional ambivalence, that is, in relation to individuals who are both loved and hated. Such indirect expressions of hatred are particularly seen in the interaction of the migrainous patient with parents, children, spouses, and employers, and revolve about the dynamic of demanded yet intolerable dependence or intimacy (see cases 62, 82, 79, and 84). A particular form of this reaction is the *emulative* migraine, in which there exists an ambivalent and malignant identification with a migrainous parent; joining the parent in illness, competing with him, hoisting him with his own migrainous petard. It seems certain that many examples of familial occurrence of migraine (as of many other illnesses) require explanation in these terms, rather than in the simplistic terms of direct inheritance (see chapter 6).

When the hostility is turned inwards, there is seen the last pattern of habitual migraine we must consider, repeated *self-punitive* attacks. Such patients are deeply masochistic, spiteful, chronically depressed, covertly paranoid, and sometimes overtly self-destructive (see case 81). The migraine rarely suffices as an expression of the inner feelings, and is likely to be accompanied by other expressions of self-hatred. These patients, in many senses, are the most deeply pathological and deeply afflicted of all; they require, as desperately as they will resist, therapeutic intervention, but this (if it is allowed by the patient) is more likely to be successful than in cases of dissociative migraine with hysterical features.

There are, of course, innumerable special uses of migraine which may cut across the broad categories we have constructed. Particularly common, and sometimes the occasion of cruel misunderstanding or punishment, are those attacks which may occur in children forced to attend schools they detest: any form of functional illness—repeated attacks of migraine, of vomiting, or of diarrhea, of asthma, or of hysterical symptoms—may serve to shield the child from some of the rigors and horrors of school life, while drawing attention to miseries which dare not, or cannot, be voiced directly.

Among famous figures who were finally liberated from intolerable conditions by such attacks must be mentioned Pope, who employed "megrim," and Gibbon, who had hysterical attacks. Gibbon later wrote of these: "The violence and variety of my complaints . . . excused my frequent absence from Westminster School . . . a strange nervous affection (painful contractions of the legs, etc.) . . . my infirmities could not be reconciled with the hours and discipline of a public seminary. . . . I secretly rejoiced in these infirmities, which delivered me from the exercises of the school and the society of my equals." Finally, on his liberation from school and his entry to Oxford, Gibbon's symptoms "most wonderfully vanished," and never returned.

We see that the emotional backgrounds of migraine may be many and various, and we would suspect that there must exist not simply *a* connection, but several types of connections, between the state of mind and the overt attack. We have already implied the probability of a major distinction in generative mechanisms by setting apart circumstantial from situational migraines. The former, we have seen, may be promptly and dramatically provoked by intense, passionate excitements—rage, terror, elation, sexual excitement, and the like. The latter, in contrast, occur in the context of emotional tensions, drives, needs, and so forth, which are chronic and have been denied direct or adequate expression: here we have recognized aggressive, destructive and libidinous drives, anxious tensions, obsessive tensions, sadistic and masochistic needs, and other behavior. We must further add that these chronic emotional needs and tensions are frequently repressed and remote from consciousness. Thus we might wonder, from the start, whether such circumstantial migraines are best considered as *reactions to* overwhelming emotion, and situational migraines, as *expressions of* chronic, repressed, emotional drives.

Thus a rage migraine may be regarded as a complex but stereotyped reaction to rage, in patients who experience this. The earlier stages of such an attack (termed earlier the phase of "engorgement") are likely to be characterized, emotionally, by irritability and angry tension, and, physiologically, by vascular and visceral dilatation, fluid retention, scanty urine production, fecal retention, and other occurrences, the symptoms of a generalized sympathetic discharge. The patient is stuffed, impacted, and bloated with anger. The resolution of the attack may proceed by crisis (brief forceful vomiting, sudden passage of flatus and feces, sneezing, etc.), or by lysis (diuresis, diaphoresis, epiphora, etc.). Thus the rage of such attacks is expressed in plethora, and discharged with a sudden visceral ejaculation (analogous to an oath or a blow), or a slow secretory catharsis (analogous to weeping). The expression of emotion proceeds by direct nervous action; it does not depend upon any intermediate conception, any conscious or unconscious symbolism uniting the affect and the physical manifestation. The symptoms of such a migraine, in Freud's terms, have no "meaning," no complex signification in the mind. Migraines of this type originate, as must all primitive reactions, in a region where emotional experience and its physiological counterparts are continuous and coextensive.

We cannot, however, construe situational migraines in terms as elementary as these, for these arise, not as expressions of acute emotional disturbance, but as expressions of chronic, and usually repressed, emotional needs. They are not simply reactions to emotion. They cannot be considered apart from their remote antecedents and effects. They have *functions*; they do *work*; they fill a dramatic role in the emotional economy of the individual; they perform, with greater or smaller success, a task of emotional equilibration, and as such are analogous to dreams, hysterical formations, and neurotic symptoms. If migraines are put to a special use, they must have a particular *meaning* for the patient; they must stand for something; they must allude to something; they must represent something. Thus it will be possible for us to approach a migraine not only as a physical event, but as a peculiar form of symbolic drama into which the patient has translated important thoughts and feelings. Thus, the particular interest of situational migraines, and their special strategic value to the patient, is that *they represent biological reactions which can double as symptomatic acts or conversion symptoms*.

Freud suggested that the symptoms of a (physical) neurosis may act as the starting point or nucleus of hysterical fabrications. We envisage that an analogous evolution may occur with the symptoms of a migraine, the initial physical symptoms becoming associated with specific emotional needs and fantasies, and thus assuming a second, symbolic, status. But a migraine is not in itself a hysterical artifice: its symptoms are real and rooted in physiological reactions. The language of hysteria is arbitrary and personal, and corresponds only to a moral, imaginative image of the body, and not to any physiological representation. In hysteria, the symbol is translated directly into a symptom: thus an arm which is, in fantasy, murderous, may be inhibited or punished by paralysis; but the hysterical paralysis does not correspond to any neurological deficit. In migraine, the symptoms are fixed and bounded by physiological connections; but its symptoms can constitute, as it were, a bodily alphabet or protolanguage, which may secondarily and subsequently be used as a symbolic language.

Thus, we must interpret situational migraines as if they were palimpsests, in which the needs and symbols of the individual are inscribed above, and yet in terms of, the subjacent physiological symptoms. Such an interpretation crosses the definitions of both conversion symptoms and vegetative neuroses, and in so doing makes the use of either term inadequate.

What starts as a direct action of the nervous system becomes, by degrees, a "serviceable associated action": what starts as the physical aspect of an emotion becomes, insensibly, an allusion to, or token of, the entire affective situation. The reactions of the body contain the potential of a primitive bodily language—in migraine, a set of inner gestures, autonomic postures, analogous to involuntary facial expressions and motor gestures. Much that Freud has said concerning the symbolism of dreams could be applied to the primitive physical symbolism of migraines. Freud sees the symbolism of dreams as archaic and universal, innate rather than individually acquired, and as representing the regressive use of "an ancient but obsolete mode of expression." Similarly, and perhaps more plausibly, the symptoms of migraine and of many other psychosomatic syndromes, in their symbolic employment, may be seen as a reversion to an ancient and universal mode of expression—a primordial language of the body—implicit in the structure and functioning of the nervous system, and available for use when required.

We have attempted to define, in the present section and its predecessor, some of the strategic functions of migraine. We have speculated that a hierarchy of determinants may be involved, from the most general reflex-reactivity of the organism, through a variety of physiological idiosyncrasies, to the most specific conversion mechanisms of the individual patient. We have postulated that if the foundations of migraine are based on universal adaptive reactions, its superstructure may be constructed differently by every patient, in accordance with his needs and symbols.

Thus we can now answer, in principle, the dilemma posed earlier, as to whether migraine is innate or acquired. It is *both*: in its fixed and generic attributes it is innate, and in its variable and specific attributes it is acquired. In an analogous manner, the universal "deep grammar" of all languages is innate (Chomsky), while every particular language is learned.

Walking, at its most elementary level, is a spinal reflex, but is elaborated at higher and higher levels until, finally, we can recognize a man by the way he walks, by *his* walk. Migraine, similarly, gathers identity from stage to stage, for it starts as a reflex, but can become a creation.

Part IV

THERAPEUTIC APPROACHES to MIGRAINE

Introduction

It could be maintained that with the clarification of the nature of migraine, so far as we have been able to accomplish this, our task is finished, and that it would be a work of supererogation to provide a glossary of "treatments." Treatment, it might be said, is *implicit* in what has already been passed. One may write a treatise on aphasia without the need to discuss speech therapy. But our subject is not strictly comparable with this: migraine is common, inflicts widespread suffering or incapacity, tends to recurrence, is benign, and is peculiarly prone to misunderstanding or mistreatment, both by patients and physicians.

We have endeavored, in the preceding portions of this essay, to present a coherent and logically consistent picture of the biology of migraine, and much of the therapeutic approach will be dictated by the considerations already implied. But medicine cannot be reduced to coherent and logically consistent terms—it is dependent on innumerable variables and intangibles, on "magic," and above all on the trusting relationship between physician and patient.

13

General Measures in the Management of Migraine

Whoever . . . sees in illness a vital expression of the organism, will no longer see it as an enemy. In the moment that I realize that the disease is a creation of the patient, it becomes for me the same sort of thing as his manner of walking, his mode of speech, his facial expression, the movements of his hands, the drawings he has made, the house he has built, the business he has settled, or the way his thoughts go: a significant symbol of the powers that rule him, and that I try to influence when I deem it right.

—Groddeck

We have observed that roughly a tenth of the population suffer from common migraines, a fiftieth of the population from classical migraines, and a minute proportion from certain rare migraine variants (migrainous neuralgia, hemiplegic migraine, etc.). A further fraction of the population, not inconsiderable, experience migraine equivalents and isolated auras, but their numbers have not been estimated since their symptoms are generally the subject of misdiagnosis. Although headache is the commonest complaint presented to the practicing physician, it is clear that only a small fraction of the migrainous population actually seek medical help.

The physician must function first as diagnostician, then as healer or adviser. He has two diagnostic tasks: the identification of the complaint that is presented to him, and the elucidation of its causes and determinants. Let us assume that he has listened to the patient, perhaps observed an attack, undertaken all investigations he considers reasonable, and assured himself that the patient's problem is indeed one of recurrent migraines. The initial history will suffice, in some cases, to delineate the pattern of attacks and their chief causes; this is likely to obtain if the problem is one of periodic migraine (attacks regularly recurring, usually at intervals of two to eight weeks, irrespective of the mode of life), or one of circumstantial migraine (in which the attacks have been clearly associated with specific provocative circumstances—excitement, exhaustion, alcohol, etc.). There will remain a large and severely afflicted group of patients who suffer very frequent attacks without easily defined antecedents, and such patients may have to be seen repeatedly, and studied carefully, before the determinants of their migraine are exposed. Two auxiliary measures may be of particular value in clarifying the patterns and determinants of repeated migraines: the keeping of two calendars (a migraine calendar and a general diary of daily events), which may reveal unsuspected circumstances as provocative of attacks, and (if deemed proper by the physician) the interviewing of close relatives who may provide invaluable information.

The physician becomes a therapeutic figure for the patient, whatever he says, whatever he does. He may see the patient once, a dozen times, or (if he is a psychiatrist) a thousand times. He may provide advice, support, or analysis, but whatever he elects to do, his relationship to the patient is preeminent. His authority, his sympathy, and the countless intangible and largely unconscious bonds which are forged in an effective doctor-patient relationship, are as important as the sense or otherwise of anything he says and does. This relationship, then, is central in the management of all patients with functional disease.

The question of *drugs* is likely to be raised at the outset, reluctantly, hopefully, or peremptorily. Innumerable drugs have been used in the treatment of migraine, many of which are successful, and a very few of which are specific (see chapter 14), and attitudes to drugs, on the part of both patient and physician, may be extremely varied. It is cruel and pointless to deny medication to an acutely suffering patient, but it is another matter altogether to tout any form of drug therapy as the sole treatment of severe, frequently recurring migraines. In the end it is up to the doctor.

The general therapeutic measures which have value for migraine patients are threefold: the avoidance of circumstances known to be provocative of attacks, the promotion of good general health, and, finally, social and psychotherapeutic measures. The first two of these may be considered together.

General Measures and Avoidance of Provocative Circumstances

One of the traditional roles of the physician is to tell the patient not to worry, take a holiday, get enough exercise, not stay up too late, and so on, and this type of advice has been given to migraine patients, with varying success, since the time of Hippocrates. Thus, Aretaeus, writing in the second century, made the following recommendations for epileptic and migrainous patients:

Promenades long, straight, without tortuosities, in a well-ventilated place, under trees of myrtle and laurel. . . . It is a good thing to take journeys . . . exercises should be sharper, so as to induce sweat and heat . . . cultivate a keen temper, without irascibility.

Liveing (1873), recognizing that migraine is no respecter of social classes, provided memorable images of two groups of people driven to migraine by the circumstances of their lives. One group suffered from

the exhaustion which is produced by a poor and insufficient diet . . . and in women by too frequent suckling or child-bearing . . . excessive hours of labor, or occupations which entail a close confinement in the unwholesome and ill-ventilated workshops and dwellings of our crowded towns . . .

For these, the poor of London, Liveing would provide better living conditions, an adequate diet, and tonics—but alas! they are beyond his reach, for social reform must precede medicine. The second group of people prone to migraine were of a different class, students and professional men, engaged in

the struggle for competence and professional position . . . the pressure and responsibilities of business, the competition and excitement of commercial speculation . . . or breaking down under the accumulating weight of family cares . . .

For *these* Liveing would recommend less ambition, less driving, more moral and emotional ease. Such advice is easily given, but is never taken. Alvarez, at the present time, has declared: "Better far perhaps is a healthy, happy rancher, than a headache-ridden professor!" but remains himself a headache-ridden professor.

Dutifully we exhort our patients, in words which have hardly changed from Aretaeus to Alvarez, and which must be construed, for the most part, as so much wasted breath. We are on firmer ground if we can counsel patients in the avoidance of specific circumstances provocative of migraine. There are countless such circumstances (many were listed in chapter 8), and it is a test of the physician's acumen to pinpoint as many as possible.

Some such patients are sensitive to flickering light of certain frequencies, and need to have their television sets adjusted. Some patients cannot tolerate a missed meal, and others cannot tolerate a heavy meal. Some cannot take more than a single drink without risking a migraine. Some cannot tolerate loss of sleep, while others, conversely, will profit from rationing of sleep. In these and similar cases, the patient will learn that he faces a choice, to avoid the provocative circumstance or risk a migraine. But in the most important category of all, those patients in whom rage or other violent emotions may precipitate a migraine, the choice is not open. As John Hunter observed, with regard to his own attacks of angina which were precipitated by exertion or emotion: "A man may resolve never to move from his chair, but he cannot resolve never to be angry."

Supportive and Psychotherapeutic Measures

Wolff (1963), in his excellent and full discussion of the psychotherapeutic approaches to migraine patients (a discussion whose scope is limited only by the fact that all Wolff's patients, like himself, exhibited the "migraine personality"), makes the point that medical attention which is too cursory is disastrous, and an important cause of allegedly "intractable" migraine.

One must appreciate that elimination of the headache may demand more in personal adjustment than the patient is willing to give. It is the role of the physician to bring clearly into focus the cost to the patient of his manner of life. The subject must then decide whether he prefers to keep his headache or attempt to get rid of it.

Wolff's statement stresses the limitations, as Groddeck questions the propriety, of the physician who undertakes to treat psychosomatic illness. Both are concerned, implicitly, with the reality of the patient's "choice"—to hold or relinquish his symptoms. Thus we come, finally to a definition of the aim of therapy.

This cannot be put in simplistic formulae of "cure" but must be conceived as a strategy individually plotted for each particular patient, an attempt to find and secure the "best" *modus vivendi* for him. This is a matter upon which there may exist a profound, if unconscious, disagreement between the patient and his physician. We must speak of the extent to which certain patients—a minority, but an important and often deeply incapacitated group of patients—may be *attached* to their symptoms, in *need* of them; the extent to which such patients may *prefer* the migraine way of life, with all its torments, to any alternative which is left open to them.

Case 18

In chapter 2 (p. 44) the story was given of a young man who had classical migraines every Sunday, which were aborted very successfully with drugs, but were then replaced by asthmas. *At this point,* therefore, I said to him: "It looks as if you may need to be ill every Sunday, whether it's migraines, or asthmas, or whatever. Do you think this is possible? Are you prepared to consider it?" He was prepared, and we then spent half a dozen valuable sessions together, examining the need for illness in his life, and the "economic" role which his Sunday migraines were playing. The value of this discussion was shown by the improvement, and finally the disappearance of his migraines, and this without any further use of drugs. He became able to *enjoy* Sundays, and lost the need to be ill.

We remarked, in the last chapter that "conversion," or, in more general terms, the use of indirect physical means and illnesses to express thwarted drives must be considered as a perpetual potential in all of us, and we stressed Deutsch's wise comment: "human beings would be most unhappy or would take far more flight into a neurosis if they could not fall sick from time to time." There are very few patients with extremely severe, unremitting migraines facing intolerable external or internal situations. We have already implied that in such patients severe migraines may either coexist with severe neuroses, or occur in their place. The attempt to dislodge severe habitual migraines in a pathologically unconcerned or hysterical personality (case 80) may force the patient to face intense anxieties and emotional conflicts which are even less tolerable than the migraines. The physical symptoms, paradoxically, may be more merciful than the conflicts they simultaneously conceal and express. We may suspect this to be the case by observation of the personality and the symptoms, and we may verify that it is the case, on occasion, by the eruption of neurotic anxiety and conflict which may follow any therapeutic attempt to disturb the *status quo*. In such cases, migraines may fill the same paradoxical role, and be invested with the same unconscious ambivalence, as severe neurotic symptoms—they defend the personality, and offer certain advantages and securities, while preventing its expansion and freedom of action: the double role of city walls. Illness in such cases, to paraphrase the words of Groddeck, is both a friend and an enemy, and will only retreat if radically new choices can be offered to the patient.*

---

*Essentially the same point is made by Freud with regard to the management of neurotic symptoms and illness: "Although it may be said . . . that he has taken 'flight into illness,' it must be admitted that in many cases the flight is fully justified, and the physician who has perceived this state will silently and considerately retire. . . . Whenever . . . advantage through illness is at all pronounced, and no substitute for it can be found in reality, you need not look forward very hopefully to influencing the neurosis through your therapy" (1920, p. 391).

14

Special Measures in the Management of Migraine

Many patients, and not a few physicians, perpetually await the appearance of a definitive *wonder drug* for the specific treatment of migraine, and many new drugs introduced upon the market are greeted as such with rapture, and promoted at the expense of all existing remedies. Readers who have opened this book at this point, its last chapter, may be assured that there have never been any such wonder drugs, and never will be; readers who have reached this point by following the course of this book will appreciate the reasons for this. The specific treatment of migraine, unlike that of Parkinsonism, is a matter of trial and choice from among a considerable number of drugs which act on specific mechanisms in the nervous system, allied to symptomatic treatment, to the use of accessory drugs, and—not least—of important measures other than pharmacological ones.

The uncertainty of drug treatment, and the unpredictability of outcome, was very well known to the older physicians. Thus Willis, in 1672, wrote of "this contumacious and rebellious Disease . . . deaf to the charms of every Medicine," and Gowers stressed that "Measures that do good in one case will fail in another, apparently quite similar."

Among the drugs that Gowers lists, and recommends—subject to the proviso that no two cases are the same, and that trial and error, rather than dogma, is the only proper guide—are *bromides* (the favorite sedative of Victorian times), *ergot*, *nitroglycerine*, and *cannibis* (in Gowers' day, recommended as a tincture). And whatever drugs are taken, Gowers notes, are liable to be useless unless combined with *general* measures: "During the attack absolute rest is essential. . . . All strong sensory impressions should be avoided."

Having spoken of more exotic and "medical" substances, Gowers endorses the popular remedies: "Strong tea and coffee are popular remedies, and occasionally give some distinct relief, which may also be obtained from a few grains of *caffeine*."

The drinking of strong coffee, indeed, was advocated by Willis, as being the *only* "medicine" worth recommending to all patients. Little has changed in 300 years!

In the original edition of this book, I went painstakingly through all the medications, and their measures, which had been recommended throughout history for sufferers from migraine, and dwelt in particular detail on the use of such current measures as *ergotamine* preparations and *methysergide* (which were particularly used [and even "pushed"] in a migraine clinic I once worked in). I will not repeat them here, because I now think, on the basis of a much longer and more varied experience, that *the vast majority of migraine attacks, and migraine sufferers, may be treated quite simply, and without recourse to complex (and potentially dangerous) drugs*.

Thus, instead of the long itemizations and evaluations of specific medications which I provided ten years ago (to which there is only a single major item addition provided by work in the seventies, namely propranolol, see below), I am now disposed to simplify this chapter, and speak of treatment for the *vast majority*, first; and, only then, of treatment for the *small minority*.

First, since 1970, I have had occasion to see numbers of more "ordinary" and "typical" migraine patients—rather than the "hopeless cases" and "medical failures" of whom I once saw so many—and I have become much more optimistic about the treatment of migraine. Second, I have emerged from the peculiar atmosphere of a "migraine clinic" into my own practice, and can now see, in retrospect, that though such a clinic afforded me an incomparable opportunity for a very intensive and concentrated experience of the varieties and complexities of migraine, it tended to impose its own "mood" and values upon me—which, in the United States, at least, is one of over-medication, over-investigation, and over-interference generally, coupled with an insufficient sense of the patient as an individual, and a responsible adult and agent with regard to his own welfare. Third, my own practice and orientation, though making use of whatever knowledge or understanding I may have as a neurologist and psychologist, has moved strongly toward that of the general practitioner, and strongly *away* from a medicine dominated by specialists.

This altered experience, and altered perspective, makes me feel I should revise this last chapter of my book—in the direction of optimism and simplicity, and of speaking to the patient, and his own general practitioner—for I now think that specialists (and "speciality clinics") should play only a small part in the care of migraine patients—although, of course, they have their uses:

> The specialist has his function
> but, to him, we are merely banal examples of
> what he knows all about. The healer I have faith in is
> someone I've gossiped
>
> and drunk with before I call him to touch me,
> someone who admits how easy it is to misconsider
> what our bodies are trying to say, for each one
> talks in a local
>
> dialect of its own that can alter during
> its lifetime . . .
>
> —W. H. Auden

The Vast Majority

We said in the last chapter that there was only one cardinal rule: one must always *listen* to the patient; and, by the same token, the cardinal sin is *not listening*, ignoring. Prior to any and all specific approaches, there must be this general approach, the establishment of a relation, a communication with the patient, so that patient and physician *understand* each other. A relationship, moreover, in which the patient is not entirely passive and compliant, believing and doing what he is told, and taking what is "ordered." Any such relation, which degrades the patient while exalting the physician, is a travesty of authority, and essentially malign, leading inevitably to a regression and a breakdown of trust.

The history of "treatments" for migraine is largely a story of medical "overkill" and patient exploitation, and the first thing to be understood by the patient, if and when the time comes for him to seek medical advice, is to insist on a full and careful *discussion* between himself and his physician, a discussion which defers to the special knowledge and skill of the latter, but is none the less a discussion between one adult and another. The wise physician will *wish* to be conservative, knowing as he does the wisdom of the body, and the natural tendency toward resolution seen in migraine—and similar disorders. He will be *against* massive "intervention" and "fussing-around," knowing (as Hippocrates did) that this is not only inane but counterproductive and may complicate the situation and *delay* its resolution.

The vast majority of migraine attacks, by virtue of the fact that they move toward resolution, after running their course of so many hours, require nothing more than the simplest measures to make these hours bearable: namely, strong tea (or coffee), rest, darkness and silence. The simplest of analgesics—aspirin, or something comparable—will take the edge off the pain in a majority of attacks; and with this diminution of the pain, there is likely to follow a diminution of nausea and other symptoms, if present (apparently by "sympathy" within the body, so that a return to health or 'valescence' of one affected organ will lead the way to a 'convalescence' of them all).

By the same token, any measure, taken for any one symptom, can help dissipate them all. If nausea is intense, an anti-emetic will help; and help *not only* the nausea, but the headache as well. A very mild sedative—a little phenobarbital, librium or valium (the equivalent of Gowers' bromides) will tend to alleviate *all* the pathological excitements—the pounding head, the irritability, the restlessness, the anxiety—and allow the fastest possible resolution of attacks.

In the original edition of this book I spoke much of ergotamine and other drugs that can *abort* an attack, just as there are physiological measures (exercise, sleep, etc.) which may also achieve this. I am now less certain of the wisdom of aborting attacks, and instead of advising such drugs straightaway, I would have the patient consider the pros and cons of letting the attack develop naturally. The following case history will illustrate this:

Case 75

A middle-aged professor, of fiery temperament, who tends to get classical migraines on Friday afternoons, following his inspired and stormy teaching sessions. He has scarcely time to rush home from these before scotomata and other symptoms make their appearance, followed within minutes by violent hemicrania, nausea, and vomiting. If these symptoms are *endured*, they run their course and resolve in three hours, leaving a wonderful sense of refreshment, and almost of rebirth. If, on the other hand, they are *aborted* (as they may be by ergotamine, exercise, or sleep), there is a persistent malaise throughout the entire weekend. Thus this patient is presented with a *choice*: to be violently ill for three hours, and then perfectly well; or to be vaguely ill and wretched for two to three *days*. Since realizing his situation, he has given up the use of all abortive measures, finding a severe but brief migraine altogether preferable to a mild but greatly extended one.

Somewhat similar considerations—and it is not clear whether they should be seen as physiological, psychological, moral, or economic—apply to *fighting* attacks (see self-perpetuation of migraines, pp. 183–184). Nobody has an attack lasting two to three *days*, by and large, unless they "ask" for it; and the commonest way of "asking" for such a protraction is to deny the attack, or its *needs*, and push on regardless as if nothing were the matter. There are, of course, situations when one *has* to do this: when one cannot afford the time off, the rest, for a migraine attack. But in most cases one can and indeed *should*; and discretion is very much the better part of valor, here.

Indeed this is true even if one has chosen the path of aborting an attack. This economic and biological point is well stressed by Wolff:

Every administration of ergotamine should be followed by rest in bed for a period of not less than two hours. The desirability of this cannot be overstated, because the biological purpose of the attack is defeated if the patient immediately resumes activity. If suitable relaxation and rest in bed is neglected after the abortion of an attack with ergotamine, headaches may actually occur with increased frequency.

One must work *with* one's biology, not against it; or one's biology will retaliate with a vengeance. One cannot deny nature, or expel it—at least in such matters as the treatment of migraine.

It might be said that such an attitude is one of "quietism" not aggression, and it is up to doctors (and medicine) to *be* aggressive, not "quiet." One may indeed say that there are here two philosophies, two schools, two *moods* of medical thought—one patient, the other impatient, in relation to nature. The former lets ailments run their course, doing what it can to make the patient comfortable, but only entering decisively if and when the right moment (*kairos*) occurs. This was precisely the mode of Hippocrates—and, as such, brought him into opposition with the "modernists" of his time (I speak of the fifth century B.C.), who felt that one should be constantly hovering round the patient, doing this, doing that, checking, pestering, intervening.

It should be clear that my own preference is for patience, not pestering, and that the atmosphere of a quiet and darkened room, with a very minimum of coming and going, is indeed preferable—so far as migraine is concerned—to the atmosphere of an intensive care unit, with its incessant, intrusive, almost frenetic activity.

There are different moods of medicine in different times—and different places. We fuss about the migraineur now, with injections and interventions, in a way which would have horrified Liveing, or the Victorians, and it is precisely this sort of fussing which makes migraine worse so that, paradoxically, the very intensity and incessancy of "treatment," these days, may serve to aggravate, not alleviate, the malady it seeks to help. The best migraine clinic I have seen was one where the sufferer was led, without an unnecessary movement or words, to a darkened cubicle, where he could lie down and rest, and receive a pot of tea and a couple of aspirin

The results of this simple, natural regimen, even with classical attacks of great severity, were far more impressive than anything I had seen in other clinics; and brought home to me with an overwhelming conviction that, for the vast majority of patients and attacks, the answer does not lie in ever-more-powerful drugs, and medicamental aggressiveness, but a sensitive feeling for suffering, and nature; a deep sense of the healing power of nature itself (*vis medicatrix naturae*), and the humility which seeks to woo nature, but never to bully it:

"Healing,"
Papa would tell me,
"is not a science,

> but the intuitive art
> of wooing nature."
>
> —W. H. Auden

The management of most migraines then, after an initial and reassuring consultation with the doctor, is very much a matter of self-help—common sense, aided by a few simple drugs, which are available over the counter, and need no prescription.

The basic drugs are caffeine, simple painkillers, and anti-emetics. Caffeine is available in standard sizes (50 mg, 100 mg, etc.)—or, more pleasantly, in coffee or tea. If these irritate the stomach, of course, they should not be taken. There are a variety of simple painkillers beside aspirin and phenacetin—if these need to be avoided because of special sensitivities, paracetamol is very safe, and available pure or in compound preparations. Nausea ranks equal with headache in frequency, and is sometimes much less tolerable than pain. There are a variety of drugs which are effective against it—most in the cyclizine or buclizine group. Codeine, of course, is notably stronger as a painkiller than aspirin, or other remedies, without being in the potency range of the opiates and narcotics; it is a prescription drug when taken "neat" in substantial doses, but may be obtained over the counter if no more than an ingredient of a compound preparation. A variety of medications, all mild in themselves, may strengthen each other's action, and produce a strong compound. This is the justification of compound proprietaries specifically aimed at migraine sufferers.

The Small Minority

A twentieth (or less) of the total migraine population have long and savage attacks which come with great frequency; and it is only these "special" patients who require special measures. I have spent the last few weeks and months speaking to general practitioners and chemists—and I find that such patients are astonishingly rare (but they constituted the majority in our special clinic in New York). The largest and busiest chemist in the neighborhood told me that they had calls for ergotamine preparations only two or three times a month, and for ergotamine injections virtually never. I found, further, that methysergide had virtually "gone out"—there had been no prescriptions in three years, and none was kept in stock. On the other hand, a number of new drugs were used steadily by a few patients—namely *clonidine* and *propranolol*—for the prevention of migraine. It was clear, however, that there was remarkably little use of such heavy prescription drugs, at most a mild traffic in over-the-counter preparations.

In the chapters on treatment in the original edition, which was addressed to my colleagues no less than to patients, I went into much detail concerning the use of heavy drugs. Here, by contrast, it is sufficient to say that *if* heavy drugs are needed, they must only be taken under medical supervision—for there is no heavy drug without the potential of side effects or hazards.

The commonest specific for severe migraine headache is *ergotamine*, which may be taken in different ways and preparations. Ergotamine would most commonly be taken by mouth, but if there were nausea and vomiting, it would have to be taken by another route—by rectal suppository, by aerosol inhalation, conceivably by injection. If ergotamine is going to work *at all*, it must be given very promptly, before the headache is established (a firmly established headache is very difficult to break, and if intolerable may require narcotic pain relievers). If a substantial dose of ergotamine has not worked in the first hour, it is not going to work, and no more should be taken. If speed of absorption is extremely important—as in migrainous neuralgias which may peak within minutes—it is probably best to take the ergotamine by inhalation (for this is virtually as fast as injection). The effects of ergotamine are made more powerful by caffeine, and their occasionally nauseating effects may be countered by barbiturates or cyclizine.

Since the serotonin antagonist *methysergide*, which I frequently used and spoke of at great length, has practically gone out, I see no point in dwelling on its varied effects. I do not imply that the drug is no longer in use: there are doubtless some patients who do well on it, and need it, but such patients would be taking it under the closest supervision.

Clonidine and propranolol, both introduced in the seventies, have powerful effects on autonomic sensitivity, tending to block or inhibit excessive "swings" and erratic reactions (such, as we have seen, are characteristic of migraineurs). Thus they are not aimed, like ergotamine, at the single, secondary symptom of headache, but at the underlying nervous sensitivity which predisposes to migraine—and to a host of other hyperreactions. Both have many uses other than in the treatment of migraine, and propranolol, in particular, has strong effects on the heart. Neither drug can be obtained without prescription, and neither should be taken without close supervision. Their introduction for the prevention of migraine, however, has made life easier and pleasanter for some rare unfortunates with an extreme physiological sensitivity to migraine.

I stress "physiological," because much commoner than severe physiological (or idiopathic) migraine is the *driving* of migraine in situations of stress (see chapter 9). Sometimes this is an acute and temporary situation, and patients need support, and possibly tranquilizers, *to see them through* the crisis period. Sometimes the stress is chronic and neurotic, and perhaps complicated by a regressive "need to be ill." Patients of this latter sort may be very hard to treat, even by the most expert and devoted general practitioner. Such patients *need* special clinics, psychotherapy, and so on—and are perhaps, the only migraine patients to do so.

Patient Associations

There are in many countries, and constantly increasing, associations for various sorts of patient: Parkinsonism, muscular dystrophy—and migraine. Such associations aim to provide information, advice and support to their members—especially the sort of help which one sufferer can give another. There is much to be said for the associations in so far as they increase confidence, competence and self-help. The hidden danger is that they may encourage "professionalism" in patients, and make their obesity, their paraplegia, their migraine, or whatever, the chief preoccupation and (narcissistic) center of the patient's life.

Alternative Treatments

Gowers spoke of *cannabis* as sometimes useful in migraine. A score or more of patients have said to me that "pot" helps their migraines. Some of these are real smokers, and fond of their pot; but there are others who light up on no other occasion. I have never recommended cannabis to a patient; but if a patient tells me it benefits his migraines, I would not discommend its use. In this, as in other matters, I am essentially pragmatic; what works, works—even if it works as a placebo. And I have nothing against placebos, provided they are harmless.

I have a bias, though not an absolute one, against the use of placebos in the treatment of migraine, even though the history of its treatment, for many centuries, has largely been one of brilliantly promoted and often brilliantly successful placebos. If the charismatic Dr. X has achieved startling results by injecting patients with the cerebrospinal fluid of pregnant sea-cows, and Dr. Y by "desensitizing" patients against endogenous helium, I will not try to deflect eager patients from their healing hands. I say only that I myself am conservative in such matters.

It seems probable that most other specific treatments for migraine: allergic "desensitization"; histamine "desensitization"; antihistamines, and other treatments (described in some detail in the original edition of this book), if they have any effect, have placebo effects. They may be absurd, but they are essentially harmless.

The use of *hormones*, however, is not without danger, and is best avoided—the sole legitimate indication being the use of steroids, under strict medical supervision, for the treatment of migrainous neuralgia or cluster headache; and perhaps very occasionally in an intractable "*status migrainosus.*"

The use of surgery is controversial: obviously the wholesale extirpation of viscera and other organs, once recommended, is quite monstrous; but the excision of the affected superficial artery in cases of intractable migraine may sometimes be justified.

MODERN DEVELOPMENTS

The last decade has seen the development of "biofeedback" techniques of considerable promise and potency. Here, by using an EEG, or other physiological indicator, which can *show* the patient his own physiology (e.g., his cerebral rhythms, of which he has no direct experience), a patient may learn to control aberrant responses—in particular, abnormal autonomic reactions, such as the exaggerated vasomotor responses which underlie migraine headache.

That one may learn to intervene, in this way, and modify one's own erring or aberrant responses, is now well established. Whether such methods will constitute a widely useful, major, and revolutionary mode of therapy—as its proponents sometimes claim—is entirely unclear at this time. The *idea* of biofeedback is genuine self-help, enabling the patient to achieve active mastery and control of himself—of a physiological self which is normally outside his control. Here, in principle, the self helps the self, and does so actively, collaboratively, instead of passively with drugs. The *principle* of such a control seems to me admirable and exciting, but I have no direct knowledge of how it works in practice. The same hopes have been entertained, and the same reservations must be made with regard to the whole "new wave" of techniques for stress reduction—meditation, yoga, and the like. The *idea* is fine, but it is far from clear as to whether the complex economy of the migraine-prone individual can be permanently altered by such methods as these.

Conclusions

The actual methods by which physicians may choose, or be forced to treat their patients is, of course, infinitely varied, as are the patients themselves. There is only one cardinal rule: one must always *listen* to the patient. For if migraine patients have a common and legitimate second complaint beside their migraines, it is that they have not been listened to by physicians. Looked at, investigated, drugged, charged—but not listened to.

Sometimes rest is prescribed, sometimes activity; sometimes yielding to an attack, sometimes fighting it; sometimes accepting what appears to be a built-in migraine "fate," sometimes struggling furiously to avert or alleviate this.

And if there is no constancy, and even contradiction, with regard to general measures, this is no less so with regard to specific measures. Thus Gowers, considering all the medications used in the treatment of migraine, wrote: "Measures that do good in one case will fail in another, apparently quite similar." This was written a century ago, but is equally true today. Why is this? Why have we not found a wholly specific and efficacious medication—Medicine X—which will revolutionize the treatment of migraine, as L-

Dopa has revolutionized the treatment of Parkinsonism? And may we hope to *find* such a medicine? My own belief, perhaps I am wrong, is that the answer here is "No," and for reasons that have been demonstrated throughout the whole book. There are, I think, two *kinds* of reason, which make migraine rather special, and its treatment, therefore, both delicate and challenging.

The first is physiological: There does not seem to be any single, invariable mechanism for the production of migraines. A migraine is a highly distinctive physiological event, and yet it is one that may be reached in a variety of ways. This, one might say, is equally true of epilepsy, of seizures, and yet one has the anticonvulsants, which dampen the convulsive irritability of the brain. But the organic irritability that predisposes to migraine seems to be of a much more general sort, and one that is intimately related to all the vital functions and autonomic controls of the body, and these one cannot alter with impunity (hence the special care needed with, and the potential dangers attending to, any use of the powerful new autonomic blockers we now have).

The second reason is that though a migraine is a physiological event, it is not *just* a physiological event, but one that tends to be strongly related to, and determined by, the affected *individual*—his character, his "needs," his circumstances, and his mode of life. Thus it is insufficient to look for purely physiological remedies, when what one may have to remedy, if it can be remedied, is a whole way of life, a whole life.

There is a tendency, increasingly, to reduce Medicine to medicines; to reduce, and to regard as irrelevant or "old-fashioned," any personal attention to the patient, and to treat, in a purely mechanical way, his physiological disorders. This is the *mood* of our harried, hurried, drug-hungry, Modern Medicine. But it is a mood that is hostile to the proper treatment of migraine—or, as one should say, to the treatment of migraine *patients*. For it is not the migraine, but the *patient*, who needs treatment. The proper treatment of migraine, then, although it will make the fullest use of whatever new discoveries and new techniques become available, must always turn and return to the affected *individual*, and find its heart in an "old-fashioned," *personal* attention.

This was always the central motto and message of Hippocrates, the Father of Medicine: that one not treat the disease, but the diseased individual; that though the doctor must be knowledgeable and expert about diseases, his final care, his concern, must be for the affected, suffering patient. This then, whether defined by Hippocrates or Groddeck, remains the central, eternal role of the physician, and of the human, humane Medicine which, ideally, he embodies. He must understand not only the disease but the patient, and through this be his guide and companion. The physician must, indeed, have Authority; and the patient, likewise, have Faith; there is not just a technical but a moral relation between them; but this will speedily become empty or corrupt if it is not based on a genuine, deeply-founded understanding.

It is neither a technique nor a "treatment" which the physician finally gives, though his giving must include techniques and treatments. What must finally be given is understanding—and courage: an *attitude* that is life-affirming, in face of disease. The patient requires *strength*, so that he can stand up alone; and then, and only then, can he dispense with the physician, because in self-understanding, self-help, he can now be physician to himself. Thus Medicine, which may first need to come from others, from the outside, must activate an inner power, a Healing Will, in the patient, and when this occurs (and one can only hope it occurs!) one's migraines, one's illnesses, lose their baleful sting, and one is firmly set on the road to life and health. One may, indeed, continue to have attacks, on occasion; and to fall back, regressively, from time to time; but one has firmly and decisively taken the upper hand; one has risen, by will and courage, *above* one's condition. Through much pain, much suffering, endured with firm fortitude, one may achieve that transcendence, which Nietzsche calls "The Great Health."

Epilogue

"The Long Road"

We have traveled a long road, with unexpected views and detours, through Migraine Land, and now we have come to the end of our journey.

For every patient with migraine there is A Long Road, and a Short Cut. The Short Cut is a diagnosis, a pill, a pat on the head. It takes all of five minutes. There is nothing wrong with this. The only thing is—it usually doesn't work. Hence the necessity, for many patients, to take The Long Road. The Long Road is the road of understanding—an understanding of the heart no less than the mind. For, as Aretaeus stressed, two thousand years ago, migraine is an illness ". . . by no means mild." And added to the miseries of the affliction itself, are the multiplying miseries of perplexity and fear: "Fear of this disease," writes Montaigne, "used to terrify you, when it was unknown to you."

For such patients, then, who are not only miserably afflicted, but ignorant, perplexed, and fearful as well, it is imperative to take The Long Road, to acquire the needed knowledge and courage, so that he may know and face what manner of thing he has.

Such a journey is scarcely to be accomplished alone; it needs a guide, a physician, or a physicianly book. This book aims to be such a guide, to guide the patient, and those who care for him, through the strange and riddling landscapes of Migraine; not merely its phenomena, which are infinitely diverse, but all the ways in which it affects, and is affected by, the life of each patient. With such a guide, a physicianly *Baedeker*, by one's side, one can set out with a clearer head and a bolder heart on that Long Road of *self-exploration* which the affliction of migraine, more than any other, seems to warrant and need.

The end of one journey is the start of another; where the writer stops the reader begins. I have tried to stimulate, to provoke, to question, to explore, to open a discourse, to open a door, on what is so often a dark and secret world. I do not have, and do not promise, any answers—I question. The answers must be found by the patient himself.

Glossary of Case Histories

Note: The above case histories are quoted *in extenso* in the text. Other case histories are alluded to more briefly, and reference to these must be sought in the Index.

Glossary of Terms

Acetylcholine   Naturally occurring "neurotransmitter," tending to serve parasympathetic and inhibitory systems, and thus antagonistic to those served by adrenalin and dopamine.

Adrenalin and Nor-adrenalin   Naturally occurring "neurotransmitters" in the nervous system, especially serving sympathetic and excitatory activity.

Agnosia   Inability to perceive through inability of the brain-mind to relate, or integrate, the components of perception. This is neither a paralysis nor a hysterical disorder, but a specific disturbance of higher brain functions.

Amusia   An alteration or deprivation in the perception of music— either in the perception of melody, or of tonality (see *Aphasia*).

Analeptic   Exciting the nervous system (*cataleptic*, strictly, would be depressing the nervous system. Tranquilizers and mood-changers are sometimes called *neuroleptics*).

Anesthesia   A complete deprivation of sensation and feeling: see also *Paresthesia* which are distortions of sensation and feeling.

Aneurysm, Angioma   Rare abnormalities of blood vessels, which may, very rarely, cause migrainelike symptoms. An *aneurysm* is a thinned-out, balloonlike swelling. An *angioma* is a tumorlike cluster of abnormal blood vessels. Properly speaking an angioma is a malformation—not a tumor.

Angioneurotic edema Swelling of the face and scalp tissues, occasionally the tongue: sometimes allergic, sometimes "nervous," sometimes seen in a migraine.

Angor animi Fear for the soul, sense of imminent dissolution, overwhelming dread and conviction of death. A peculiar and terrible form of fear, perhaps only seen with organic disturbances (migraine, angina, etc.)

Aphasia Inability, or diminished ability, to understand or use language (the former being a "receptive," the latter an "expressive" aphasia, either of which may occur independently of the other). The "three As"—apraxia-agnosia-aphasia—are not uncommon in migraine aura, at least to a mild degree (see chapter 3).

Apraxia Inability to act through inability of the brain-mind to place in relationship, or synthesize, the components of the act. This is neither a paralysis nor a hysterical disorder, but a specific disturbance of higher brain functions.

Atonia, Hypotonia, Hypertonia, and so on. Absent, diminished, or increased muscle tone. (Muscle tone is usually increased in the early, tense phases of migraine, and reduced or collapsed in the exhausted, late phases.)

Aura This term is now used for the many weird and wonderful symptoms which commonly precede the headache of migraine—and frequently replace it altogether. The word *aura* was first used by Pelops, the master of Galen, who was struck by the phenomenon with which many attacks begin. The sensation having been described to him by patients as "a cold vapor," he suggested that it might really be such, passing up the vessels then believed to contain air. Hence he named it "spirituous vapor" in Greek.

Automatism A trancelike state in which a person may perform simple habitual actions, or behave repetitively and automatically, without any consciousness or recollection afterward.

Autonomic (vegetative) That part of the nervous system, centered in the brain, but spreading into nerves and nerve plexuses all over the body, which regulates the tone and activity of blood vessels, glands, involuntary muscles, and so forth, and which is wholly automatic and unconscious in its functions. It is sometimes called the vegetative nervous system. One may say that it is disturbances of autonomic or vegetative function, above all, which dominate the picture of common migraine. Common migraine is essentially a vegetative disorder (see also *Sympathetic/parasympathetic*).

Borborygmi An onomatopoeic word, referring to noises and spasms in the distended, flatulent gut.

Bradycardia See *Tachycardia*.

Cataplexy A sudden loss of muscular tone, sometimes brought on by sudden emotion, or migraine: sometimes associated with narcolepsy, sleep paralysis, and the like.

Catarrh Excessive secretion from the nose (or, indeed, anywhere else: thus older physicians might speak of a bladder catarrh, etc.).

Cephalalgia (usually shortened to cephalgia) Head pain—nothing more.
   Similar words in the older literature—gastralgia (stomach pain), pectoralgia (chest pain). The only "algia" commonly spoken of now is *neuralgia*.

Chemosis An inflammation and exudation at the surface of the eye, making it moist and shiny. Chemosis is very frequent in migraine attacks (see page 19).

Cholecystitis Inflammation of the gallbladder.

Chorea (literally, "dance") An odd, dancing, twitching movement, moving desultorily from one part of the body to another. Most commonly seen in certain diseases (Huntington's chorea, etc.), or in Parkinsonians treated with L-Dopa, it may sometimes occur for a few minutes in a migraine (chapter 3). Complex choreic movements have some resemblance to *tics*.

Constitution, (pre)Disposition, Diathesis Archaic but powerful general terms indicating a radical (and perhaps ineradicable) psychophysiological character or *nature*, which makes one peculiarly susceptible to migraine, or whatever else is in question. It is often implied that this character or nature is *innate*, as opposed to something learned or acquired.

Crohn's disease Regional inflammation of the small bowel or *ileum.*

"Daymare" A nightmarelike experience occurring while awake, side by side, so to speak, with normal, waking consciousness.

Depersonalization, Derealization, Ego dissolution Loss of the sense of one's self, and of one's world, or "reality" (see page 93). Common in schizophrenia, but also acute migraine, and other organic disorders.

Detumescence A subsidence, after an engorgement: as with a genital reaction, a rage, a creative furor—or a migraine.

Diaphoresis (diaphora) Sweating, especially excessive sweating.

Diathesis See *Constitution*.

Diuresis Excessive production of urine.

Dopamine Allied to adrenalin—a neurotransmitter—especially concerned with "tuning up" levels of neural activity.

Dysrhythmia (see *Electroencephalography, EEG*) A special vocabulary has grown up to describe the appearance of the brain waves, as these may be recorded by EEG. Normal brain waves are remarkably rhythmical, and regular, in appearance: a lack of proper rhythm is called a *dysrhythmia.* Excessive excitement—as in an epilepsy, or some migraine auras—may make the waves high, sharp and steep, culminating in the formulation of *spikes.* There are also characteristic changes during sleep, lethargy, inattention, and sometimes migraine.

Ecchymosis Spontaneous bruising, or suffusion of blood.

Edema Swelling of tissues, an organ, or a limb, and so forth due to abnormal accumulation of body fluids.

Ego-dissolution See *Depersonalization*.

Electroencephalography (EEG) Recording cerebral activity (brain waves) through electrodes on the scalp.

Encephalization The ascent of neural functions to higher and higher levels of the brain.

244 Glossary of Terms

Enophthalmos, Exophthalmos Sunken-eyedness, or pop-eyedness, respectively. Both may be seen during migraine attacks, and reflect alteration in the tone or tuning of eye nerves.

Epigastric Just above the stomach.

Erythema (or *rubor*) Redness.

Exudation See *Transudation*.

Field The way in which the brain maps and organizes sensations conveyed to it from the senses. Most commonly we speak of the *visual* fields. A gap, defect or hiatus in a field is a *scotoma* (see *Scotoma*). Special forms of field defect have other special names, for example, see *Hemianopia*.

Figments Half-formed, fragmentary sounds, and sights, below the level of recognizable images. Very characteristic of migraine aura, delirium and other cerebral excitements.

Forced thinking Trains of thought, reminiscence, ideas, feelings, and other occurrences which appear to be forced on one, and which one is compelled to pursue. Common in schizophrenia, but equally common in organic disturbances like migraine, epilepsy, fever, delirium.

Formication A crawling feeling, as of ants on the skin.

Genetic, Genes, and so on. Inheritance (of mental and physical traits, inheritance of constitution, and of particular diatheses, etc.) is considered to be based on one's genetic character; the constellations of hereditary particles, or *genes*, in one's make-up. Such genes, or gene groups, are described as dominant, recessive, of such-and-such penetrance, and so forth depending on their power to determine or predetermine traits.

Hebetude A *dullness* of sensation, emotion, and other feelings, often seen in the late, exhausted phases of migraine.

Hemianopia A peculiar sort of blindness, arising from disorder in the brain, in which there is loss of *half* the visual field. The lost part does not look *dark* (as in ordinary blindness), but nonexistent. Thus a person may not be aware of hemianopia (or scotoma)—not only losing the sight of one half, but also losing the *idea* of this half (see chapter 3).

Hemiplegia　Paralysis of one side, seen in strokes, tumors, and (very rarely) migraines. A hemiplegia follows upon depression or destruction of the motor areas in one half (hemisphere) of the brain. A *hemianopia*—much commoner in migraine—upon involvement of the visual areas. *Hemisensory* deficits, or *hemianesthesia* may result from involvement of the general sensory or tactile areas.

Higher integrative (or cortical) *functions*　The neuropsychological (brain-mind) functions required for the putting together of speech, complex actions, perceptions, and the like. When disturbed, we find such disorders as *agnosia, aphasia, apraxia, amusia*.

Histamine　An amine found in the nervous system and other tissues, which can serve as a transmitter of nerve impulses (see Histamine headache, chapter 4).

Homeostasis　The maintenance of physiological constancy and stability. This (according to Claude Bernard, who introduced the concept) is the "purpose" of all physiological controls, and is "the condition of a free life." In disease, and in migraine, homeostasis is disturbed, and with this diminution in stability comes a corresponding reduction in freedom of activity.

Horner's syndrome　An inhibition or paralysis of the sympathetic nerves to the eye, so the eye droops, produces tears, has a small pupil, and so on. May occur transiently in migraine, most especially migrainous neuralgia (see chapter 4).

Hypertension, Hypotension　Respectively, an unusually high or low "tension" or level of blood pressure.

Hypoglycemia　Abnormally low blood-sugar—an occasional cause or concomitant of migraine.

Ictus　A seizure, or attack of any kind. Prior to a seizure there may be *pre-ictal* excitement, and, succeeding it, *post-ictal* exhaustion (and immunity).

Idiopathy　A feeling or malady arising *on its own*, and not obviously in response to some other cause. Thus idiopathic migraines come out of the blue, while symptomatic ones may follow a Chinese meal or a rage (see chapter 7).

Induration   Inflammatory thickening.

Lacrimation   Tearing: specifically, a physiological, involuntary, nonemotional production of tears.

Laryngismus   A spasm of the larynx (compare, vaginismus, tenesmus, and similar formations).

Latent, Dormant, and so on.   Latent means "hidden," dormant "asleep." It is commonly held that one does not *acquire* migraine out of the blue, but that one may have some "latent" or "dormant" tendency to it, which is made actual, or *manifest*, under provocative conditions.

Meisosis, Mydriasis   Contraction and dilatation of pupils respectively.

Metamorphoses   Transformations. Specifically, here, the transformations of migraine into (or from) other disorders—transformations which involve *equivalence* in some sense(s) (see chapter 2).

Migraine   Derived from *hemicrania* (half head), indicating that its headache is commonly confined to either side (or sometimes, alternating sides) of the head. Despite the word, headache is *never* the sole feature of a migraine (see page 11).

Migraineur/migraineuse   A male/female sufferer from migraine.

Migralepsy   Hybrid word for a hybrid attack which combines features of both migraine and epilepsy.

Mosaic vision, Cinematic vision   In mosaic vision the sense of *spatial* articulation and continuity is lost, and one sees a flat mosaic, without spaciousness or meaning. In cinematic vision the sense of *time* is fractured, the sense of continuity, articulation, and development in time; and one sees the world as a sequence of motionless stills.

Myoclonic jerks   Violent jerks involving large portions of the body's musculature. Such jerks happen to everybody, on occasion, while falling asleep. They tend, however, to be especially common before and during some migraines.

Narcolepsy   A brief, sudden, usually dream-charged sleep, which may be of compelling power and gives little warning. Narcolepsy is often related to nightmares, sleepwalking, sleep paralysis (when one is awake, but unable to move), and other phenomena. All such sleep disorders are related to migraine.

Neuralgia   The pain of an irritated, inflamed or injured nerve. Such pains tend to be excruciatingly, wincingly violent—though often very short-lived ("lightning pains"). They are seen especially in migrainous neuralgia (chapter 4). The quality of pain is very characteristic, and quite different from that of *vascular pain* (the pain of swollen, throbbing blood vessels) and of *muscular* pain (the ache of muscles tensed, or in spasm), which are much commoner in migraine.

Neurogenic   Produced by the nervous system. Thus one may experience fever in a migraine, not due to any inflammation or infection, but purely "neurogenic."

Neuropsychological   The relation (or correlation) of altering conditions of the nervous system with altering states of perception, feeling, and of mind; the grounding of psychology in neurology and physiology. All the phenomena of migraine allow neuropsychological study, but the most wonderful such correlations are to be found in the migraine *aura* (see chapter 3).

Nor-adrenalin   See *Adrenalin*.

Oliguria   Scanty urine production.

Oneiric   Of, or belonging to, dreams.

Ophthalmoplegia   Partial or complete paralysis of eye movement—which may occur very rarely (and transiently) in migraine—due to disorder of the eyes' controls in the brain (chapter 4).

Orthostatic hypotension   Inability to maintain normal blood pressure when standing; so, liability to feel dizzy, or faint, on sudden standing.

Pancreatitis   Inflammation of the pancreas.

Paresthesia   Tingling feelings, in any part of the body produced by disorder of the nervous system. *Un*pleasant tingling may be called *dysethesia*. Other disturbances of feeling (e.g., the sensation of a tight band, of a plaster cast, of subjective heat or cold)—all disturbances of normal feeling may be called paresthesia. If the disturbances are very complex, and assume the form of images, we speak of *phantoms*. The most complex paresthesia and phantoms are only seen in migraine *aura* (see chapter 3).

Pathognomonic   Symptoms and signs considered wholly characteristic—or *diagnostic*—of a particular disorder.

Phosphenes   Tiny, subjective radiances or sparks, very common in the early stages of a migraine—even commoner than full-fledged scotomata.

Photophobia, Phonophobia (literally hatred of light, hatred of sound)   The exaggerated, almost intolerable sensitivity to these which frequently occur in the course of a migraine (see pages 26–27).

Plethora   Congestion.

Prodrome (literally, "running before")   The early or inaugural features of a migraine which often serve as a warning of an impending attack.

Prosopagnosia   A specific inability to recognize *faces*—and also facial and bodily *expressions*. This may give rise to disorientation, and even depersonalization, derealization, and so on.

Pseudomigraine   Term often used for the occurrence of migraine, or migrainelike symptoms, in consequence of an anatomical abnormality in the brain (a tumor, a malformation, an aneurysm, etc.). *These are rare*. Pseudomigraines may also be called symptomatic migraines—to distinguish them from idiopathic attacks which have no such structural abnormality underlying them.

Psychophysiological   A highfalutin word for the simplest and deepest mystery in the world—the relation of "soul" and "body," and specifically, their going together in health and disease. Migraine is here portrayed as a most common and striking *psychophysiological reaction*, involving changes of attitude and mood inseparable from all the physical changes (see *Psychosomatic*; *Neuropsychological*).

Psychosomatic Physical responses to mental or emotional stimuli, for example, the occurrence of ulcers, asthma—and, of course, migraine—when these can be related to heightened emotion or stress.

Ptosis Drooping of an eyelid.

Scintillation The sort of twinkling which is very characteristic of many of the visual phenomena of migraine—especially the crescentic expanding scotomata—the twinkling of phosphenes—and of cinematic vision.

Scotoma (literally, darkness or shadow) Dramatic disturbances in vision and the visual field, taking the form of strange and often twinkling brilliances (scintillating scotomata), or strange blindnesses and absences of vision. Without doubt scotomata, of one sort or another, are the most common feature of migraine other than headache and, possibly, commoner than headache itself (see chapter 3).

Spectrum A luminous scotoma in the visual field, colored and arched like a rainbow (see chapter 3).

Splanchnic Involuntary tissues and activities of the viscera: often engorged, and increased, in the early portions of a migraine—as with vascular (and glandular) appearance and activity.

Sternutatory Provocative of sneezinglike snuff. Useful on occasion in terminating a migraine.

Stigmata Stigmata are signs or marks of disease—or, indeed, of anything else (such as the stigmata of grace—or disgrace). The term carries a signification over and above the purely medical terms "pathognomonic" and "diagnostic," indicating that the sufferer is "marked" and singled out. One might say that over and above the medical problems of having a disorder stand the problems of being *stigmatized* by it. Epileptics may be most cruelly (and unjustly) stigmatized; migraineurs, mercifully, are much less so.

Synaesthesia A "fusion" between normally distinct senses, so that sounds, for example, may be "seen," felt, and tasted (wonderfully described in *The Mind of a Mnemonist* by Luria). Probably a primitive state—may be normal in early infancy.

Syncope   A brief loss or interruption of consciousness—a blackout.

Syndrome (literally, like "concurrence" or "concourse," a *running-together*).   A key word and key concept in our understanding of migraine, or of any other medical or "organic" condition. A syndrome is an *association*, but not just a random or mechanical one (like a junk shop). It is an organic association of features which *naturally* go together, and which therefore form a sort of composite or unity. Thus we may speak of migraine syndromes, Parkinsonian syndromes, personality syndromes, as well as others. We may perceive a syndrome, or that something *is* a syndrome, long before we are able to dissect it: and classical medicine (or *nosology*) is a natural history of such syndromes—as biology is a natural history and classification of organic beings.

Sympathetic/parasympathetic   These are the two great divisions of the *autonomic* (or vegetative) nervous system (see also *Autonomic*). Actions of the sympathetic system "tone up" the organism—increasing muscular tone, blood flow to muscles, heart action, blood pressure, wakefulness, energy, and affect other functions, thus preparing the organism for work, or fight-flight (sometimes called *ergotropic*). The parasympathetic system, by contrast, is concerned with consolidation, conservation, rest—and, when active (after meals, during sleep, and in the latter part of a migraine) *reduces* energy, vigilance, heart rate, muscle tone, and so on, while increasing the activity of the viscera and glands (sometimes called *trophotropic*). There is normally a fine "tuning" or balance between these two systems—but this is grossly disturbed in a migraine.

Sympathotonic/vagotonic (see *Sympathetic/parasympathetic, Autonomic*, etc.)   Old terms, once widely used, indicating a preponderant tendency to overstimulation of the sympathetic system (which would be shown as irritability, rage, tension, etc.), or of the opposite parasympathetic or vagal system (which would be shown as weakness, collapse, withdrawal, etc.). Such abnormal sensitivities, and lack of autonomic balance, have been considered as characteristic, or common, in migraineurs.

Sympathy (literally "feeling together" or "suffering together") Often used with regard to various *organs*, in the older views of migraine, for example, the stomach suffering in sympathy with the head (see pages 3–4).

Tachycardia, Bradycardia Exceptionally rapid or exceptionally slow heart beat, respectively.

Tinnitus A high-pitched ringing sound, which may occur briefly in a migraine, sometimes accompanied by distortions in hearing, partial deafness, or vertigo. Tinnitus is the auditory equivalent of scintillations or phosphenes in sight, as formication and paresthesia are their equivalents in touch.

Transudation A passage of fluid from one compartment of the body, or one tissue, to another. Passage *out*, that is, on to, the surface of an organ or the skin, is *exudation*.

Trophic The *nutritive* functions of nerves and blood are called "trophic." If they are inadequate, we see dystrophy, or atrophy. Such changes are rare, and usually transient, in migraine, and occur in relation to extremities, such as skin, nails, hair.

Turbinates Bony structures in the nostrils, resembling little scrolls or turbans.

Uncinate seizures Epileptic seizures (or migraines) arising in the *uncus*, deep in the brain. Such attacks are characterized by strange smells, a strange feeling of "having been there before" (*déjà vu*), sometimes vivid recollections of childhood, and occasionally speech disturbances.

Urticaria Hives.

Vasovagal Having reference to the vagus nerve, and its relation to the tone of blood vessels. This is suddenly diminished in a so-called vasovagal attack (or faint).

Vertigo A sensation of spinning—very sickening and intolerable— with an acute loss of orientation and balance.

Suggested Reading

Alexander, Frans. *Psychosomatic Medicine: its Principles and Applications*. W. W. Norton & Co., New York, 1950.

———. (1948). "Fundamental Concepts of Psychosomatic Research," pp. 3–13, in *Studies in Psychosomatic Medicine: an Approach to the Causes and Treatment of Vegetative Disorders*. The Ronald Press, New York, 1948.

Alexander, F., and French, T. M. *Studies in Psychosomatic Medicine: an Approach to the Causes and Treatment of Vegetative Disorders*. The Ronald Press, New York, 1948.

Alvarez, W. C. (1959). "Some Characteristics of the Migrainous Woman." *N. Y. State J. Med.* 59:2176.

———. (1960). "The Migraine Scotoma as studied in 618 Persons." *Amer. J. Ophth.* 49:489.

Aretaeus. *The Extant Works of Aretaeus the Cappadocian*. (Francis Adam's translation: printed for the Sydenham Society.) Wertheimer & Co., London, 1856.

Balyeat, R. M. *Migraine: Diagnosis and Treatment*. J. B. Lippincott Co., Philadelphia & London, 1933.

Beaumont, G. E. *Medicine*. (6th ed.) J. & A. Churchill, London, 1952.

Bickerstaff, E. R. (1961). "Basilar Artery Migraine." *Lancet* 1:15.

———. (1961). "Impairment of Consciousness in Migraine." *Lancet* 2:1057.

Blau, J. N., and Whitty, C. W. M. (1955). "Familial Hemiplegic Migraine." *Lancet* 2:1115.

Bleuler, E. *Dementia Praecox, or the Group of Schizophrenias*. International Universities Press, New York, 1958.

Bradshaw, P., and Parsons, M. (1963). "Hemiplegic Migraine: a Clinical Study." *Quart. J. Med.* 34:65.

Burn, J. H. *The Autonomic Nervous System*. Blackwell, Oxford, 1963.

Cannon, W. B. *Bodily Changes in Pain, Hunger, Fear, and Rage*. (2d ed.) D. Appleton & Co., New York, 1920.

Critchley, MacDonald (1936). "Prognosis in Migraine." *Lancet* 1:35.

———. (1963). "What is Migraine?" *J. Coll. Gen. Pract.* 6 (supp. 4):5.

———. (1964). "The Malady of Anne, Countess of Conway: a case for commentary," pp. 91–7, in *The Black Hole and Other Essays*. Pitman Medical Publ. Co., London, 1964.

Darwin, Charles. *The Expression of the Emotions in Man and Animals*. (2d ed.) Murray, London, 1890.

Deutsch, F. *On the Mysterious Leap from the Mind to the Body*. International Universities Press, New York, 1959.

Dexter, J. (1968). Personal communication. (See p. 163.)

Dunning, H. S. (1942). "Intracranial and Extracranial Vascular Accidents in Migraine." *Arch. Neurol. Psychiat.* 48:396.

Farquhar, H. G. (1956). "Abdominal Migraine in Children." *Brit. Med. J.* 1:1062.

Fitz-Hugh, T., Jr. (1940). "Praecordial Migraine: an Important Form of 'Angina Innocens.'" *New Int. Clinics* 1 (series 3):143.

Foucault, M. *Madness and Civilization*. Random House, New York, 1965.

Freud, Sigmund (1920). *A General Introduction to Psychoanalysis*. Reprinted by Washington Square Press, New York, 1952.

Friedman, A. P., Harter, D. H., and Merritt, H. H. (1961). "Ophthalmoplegic Migraine." *Trans. Amer. Neur. Ass.* 86:169.

Fromm-Reichmann, F. (1937). "Contributions to the Psychogenesis of Migraine." *Psychoanal. Rev.* 24:26.

Furmanski, A. R. (1952). "Dynamic Concepts of Migraine: A Character Study of One Hundred Patients." *Arch. Neurol. Psychiat.* 67:23.

Gardener, J. W., Mountain, G. E., and Hines, E. A. (1940). "The Relationship of Migraine to Hypertension Headache." *Amer. J. Med. Sc.* 200:50.

Gellhorn, Ernst. *Principles of Autonomic-Somatic Integration*. University of Minnesota Press, Minneapolis, 1967.

Gibbs, F. A., and Gibbs, E. L. *Atlas of Electroencephalography*. Lew A. Commings Co., Cambridge, Mass., 1941, and Addison-Wesley Press Inc., Cambridge, Mass., 1950.

Goodell, H., Lewontin, R., and Wolff, H. G. (1954). "The Familial Occurrence of Migraine Headache: a Study of Heredity." *Ass. Research Nerv. Ment. Dis.* 33:346.

Goodman, L. S., and Gilman, A. *The Pharmacological Basis of Therapeutics*. (2d ed.) Macmillan, New York, 1955.

Gowers, W. R., Sir (1881). *Epilepsy and Other Chronic Convulsive Diseases: their Causes, Symptoms, and Treatment*. Dover Publications Reprint, New York, 1964.

———. *A Manual of Diseases of the Nervous System*. (2d ed.) J. & A. Churchill, London, 1892.

———. *Subjective Sensations of Sight and Sound: Abiotrophy, and Other Lectures*. P. Blakiston's Son & Co., Philadelphia, 1904.

———. *The Borderland of Epilepsy: Faints, Vagal Attacks, Vertigo, Migraine, Sleep Symptoms, and their Treatment*. P. Blakiston's Son & Co., Philadelphia, 1907.

Graham, J. R. (1952). "The Natural History of Migraine: Some Observations and a Hypothesis." *Trans. Amer. Clin. & Climat. Ass.* 64:61.

Greene, R. (1963). "Migraine—the Menstrual Aspect." *J. Coll. Gen. Pract.* 6 (supp. 4):15.

Groddeck, George. *The Book of the It*. (Authorized translation of Das Buch vom Es, 1923.) Random House, New York, 1949.

Hebb, D. O. "The Problem of Consciousness and Introspection" in *Brain Mechanisms and Consciousness*, edited by J. F. Delafresnaye. Charles C. Thomas, Springfield, Ill., 1954.

Heberden, William. *Commentaries on the History and Cure of Diseases*. T. Payne, London, 1802.

Heyck, H. *Neue Beiträge für Klinik und Pathogenese der Migräne*. Theime, Stuttgart, 1956.

Horton, B. T. (1956). "Histaminic Cephalgia: Differential Diagnosis and Treatment." *Proc. Mayo Clinic* 31:325.

Jackson, J. Hughlings. *Selected Writings of John Hughlings Jackson*. Edited by James Taylor. Hodder & Stoughton, London, 1931.

Janet, P. (1921). "A Case of Sleep lasting Five Years, with Loss of

Sense of Reality." *Arch. Neurol. & Psychiat.* 6:467.

Jones, Ernest. *On the Nightmare.* Hogarth Press, London, 1949.

Klee, A. *A Clinical Study of Migraine with Particular Reference to the Most Severe Cases.* Munksgaard, Copenhagen, 1968.

Konorski, Jerzy. *Integrative Activity of the Brain: an Interdisciplinary Approach.* University of Chicago Press, Chicago, 1967.

Lance, J. W., and Anthony, M. (1960). "Some Clinical Aspects of Migraine." *Arch. Neurol.* 15:356.

Lance, J. W., Anthony, M., and Hinterberger, H. (1967). "The Control of Cranial Arteries by Humoral Mechanisms and its Relation to the Migraine Syndrome." *Headache* 7:93.

Lashley, K. S. (1941). "Patterns of Cerebral Integration indicated by Scotomas of Migraine." *Arch. Neurol. Psychiat.* 46:331.

Lees, F., and Watkins, S. M. (1963). "Loss of Consciousness in Migraine." *Lancet* 2:647.

Lennox, W. G. *Science and Seizures: New Light on Epilepsy and Migraine.* Harper and Bros., New York, 1941.

Lennox, W. G., and Lennox, M. A. *Epilepsy and Related Disorders.* (2 volumes.) Little, Brown & Co., Boston, 1960.

Leroy, R. (1922). "The Syndrome of Lilliputian Hallucinations." *J. Nerv. & Ment. Dis.* 56:325.

Lippman, C. W. (1953). "Hallucinations of Physical Duality in Migraine." *J. Nerv. & Ment. Dis.* 117:345.

Liveing, Edward. *On Megrim, Sick-Headache, and Some Allied Disorders: A Contribution to the Pathology of Nerve-Storms.* Churchill, London, 1873.

Luria, A. P. *Higher Cortical Functions in Man.* Translated by Basil Haigh. Basic Books, New York, 1966.

Miller, W. R. (1936). "Psychogenic Factors in Polyuria of Schizophrenia." *J. Nerv. & Ment. Dis.* 84:418.

Milner, P. M. (1958). "Note on a Possible Correspondence between the Scotomas of Migraine and the Spreading Depression of Leão." *Electroenceph, Clin. Neurophysiol.* 10:705.

Mingazzini, G. (1926). "Klinischer Beitrag zum Studium der cephalalgischen und hemikranischen Psykosen." *Z. ges. Neurol. Psychiat.* 101:428.

Pavlov, I. P. *Lectures on Conditioned Reflexes.* Translated by W. Horsley Gantt. International Publishers, New York, 1928–41.

Penfield, W., and Perot, P. (1963). "The Brain's Record of Auditory and Visual Experience—a Final Summary and Discussion." *Brain* 86:595.

Penfield, W., and Rasmussen, T. *The Cerebral Cortex of Man*. The Macmillan Co., New York, 1950.

Peters, J. C. *A Treatise on Headache*. William Radde, New York, 1853.

Rieff, P. *Freud: The Mind of the Moralist*. Doubleday & Co., New York, 1959.

Selby, G., and Lance, J. W. (1960). "Observations on 500 cases of Migraine and Allied Vascular Headache." *J. Neurol. Neurosurg. Psychiat*. 23:23.

Selye, H. (1946). "The General Adaptation Syndrome and Diseases of Adaptation." *J. Clinic. Endocrinol*. 6:117.

Singer, Charles. "The Visions of Hildegard of Bingen" in *From Magic to Science*. Dover, New York, 1958.

Symonds, C. (1952). "Migrainous Variations." *Trans. Med. Soc. London* 67:237.

Tissot, Simon André. *An Essay on the Disorders of People of Fashion*. Translated by F. B. Lee. S. Bladon, London, 1770. See also the last volume of *Traité des nerfs et leurs maladies*, of which 83 pages are devoted to the subject of migraine. Paris, 1778–90.

Vahlquist, B., and Hackzell, G. (1949). "Migraine of Early Onset." *Acta Paediatrica* 38:622.

Weiss, E., and English, O. S. *Psychosomatic Medicine: a Clinical Study of Psychophysiological Reactions*. W. B. Saunders Co., Philadelphia & London, 1957.

Whitty, C. W. M. (1953). "Familial Hemiplegic Migraine." *J. Neurol. Neurosurg. Psychiat*. 16:172.

Whytt, Robert. *Diseases commonly called Nervous, Hypochondriac, or Hysteric*. Becket, Pond, & Balfour, Edinburgh. 1768.

Willis, Thomas. *De Morb. Convuls*. (Amstel, 1670), *De Anima Brutorum* (Oxon, 1672). First English translation (Pordage) in *Dr. Willis' practice of Physick, Being the Whole Works of that Renowned and Famous Physician*. London, 1684.

Wolff, H. G. *Headache and other Head-Pain*. Oxford University Press, New York, 1963.

I greatly regret not having made reference to J.W. Lance's accessible yet authoritative *Mechanism and Management of Headache* (Butterworth Scientific). The first edition of this was published in 1969, when the original edition of *Migraine* was already in press. Readers who desire to go more deeply into the technical aspects of the subject, or to acquaint themselves with the most important current research, are strongly recommended to consult the fourth (1982) edition of this invaluable book.

Index